Nahrung

Food

Chemie
Biochemie
Mikrobiologie
Technologie
Ernährung

Mitarbeiter-Bedingungen

1. Es werden nur solche Arbeiten angenommen, die dem Inhalt nach wertvoll und nicht an anderer Stelle veröffentlicht worden sind. Die Manuskripte bitten wir in deutscher oder englischer Sprache in Original-Maschinenschrift (keine Durchschrift) einseitig und zweizeilig, mit 4 cm breitem Rand versehen, einzureichen.
2. Die Einsendung des Manuskriptes bitten wir an die Redaktion der Zeitschrift „Die Nahrung" vorzunehmen. Eingang und Annahme der Arbeit werden dem Autor schriftlich bestätigt.
3. Am Kopf der Arbeit ist die Institution anzugeben, aus der die Arbeit stammt. Danach folgt der Titel der Arbeit. Unter dem Titel ist der Name des Verfassers (mit Vornamen-Initial) ohne Berufsbezeichnung, akademischen Grad o. ä. anzugeben. Die vollständige Anschrift der Autoren mit Namen und Titel ist im Anschluß an die Literatur anzugeben.
4. An den Anfang der Arbeit ist eine Zusammenfassung zu stellen (maximal 25 Schreibmaschinenzeilen). Sie soll neben einer kurzen Problemstellung die wichtigsten Ergebnisse enthalten und über den Inhalt der Arbeit hinreichend informieren. Angaben, für deren Verständnis in der Arbeit nachgelesen werden muß (z. B. Abkürzungen, Literaturhinweise), sind zu unterlassen. Übersetzungen der Zusammenfassung in die russische, englische bzw. deutsche Sprache sind erwünscht und werden am Schluß der Arbeit (vor dem Literaturverzeichnis) gebracht.
5. Unbedingt erforderliche Abbildungen finden Aufnahme, wenn gut reproduzierbare Vorlagen eingesandt werden. Graphische Darstellungen und Formelbilder sind sorgfältig zu zeichnen. Die Bildunterschriften sind auf einem gesonderten Blatt beizufügen. Die doppelte Darstellung von Ergebnissen in Abbildungen und Tabellen ist zu vermeiden.
6. Literaturangaben sind am Schluß der Arbeit wie folgt aufzuführen: bei Büchern unter Angabe von Autor (mit Vorname-Initial), Titel, Verlag, Verlagsort und Erscheinungsjahr; bei Zeitschriften-Aufsätzen unter Angabe von Autor (mit Vorname-Initial), Zeitschriftentitel (Abkürzungen nach TGL 20969 „Zeitschriftenkurztitel", April 1969), Bandzahl (unterstrichen), Seitenzahlen (von – bis), Erscheinungsjahr (in Klammern).
7. Für Fachausdrücke gilt die c-Schreibweise (z. B. Calcium, Glucose, Coenzym A usw.). Für die übrige Rechtschreibung ist „Der Große Duden" maßgebend. Die Redaktion behält sich eine redaktionelle Überarbeitung der angenommenen Manuskripte vor; größere Änderungen werden jedoch nur mit Einverständnis des Autors vorgenommen. Von jeder Originalarbeit erhält der Autor kostenlos bis zu 50 Stück Sonderdrucke geliefert. Ein Mehrbetrag wird berechnet. Es wird empfohlen, die Kosten vorher beim Verlag zu erfragen.

Zeitschrift „Die Nahrung"

Herausgeber: Der Direktor des Zentralinstituts für Ernährung der Akademie der Wissenschaften der Deutschen Demokratischen Republik.

Verlag: Akademie-Verlag, DDR-108 Berlin, Leipziger Str. 3 – 4; Fernruf 2236221 und 2236229; Telex-Nr. 114420; Bank: Staatsbank der DDR, Kto.-Nr.: 6836-26-20712.

Chefredaktion: Dr. Ulrich Behnke, Prof. Dr. Max Ulmann (Chefredakteur). Dr. Joachim Voigt.

Anschrift der Redaktion: Zentralinstitut für Ernährung der Akademie der Wissenschaften der DDR, DDR-1505 Bergholz-Rehbrücke, Arthur-Scheunert-Allee 114/116.

Veröffentlicht unter der Lizenznummer 1287 des Presseamtes beim Vorsitzenden des Ministerrates der Deutschen Demokratischen Republik.

Gesamtherstellung: VEB Druckerei „Thomas Müntzer", DDR-582 Bad Langensalza.

Erscheinungsweise: Die Zeitschrift „Die Nahrung" erscheint jährlich in einem Band mit 10 Heften. Bezugspreis je Heft 18, – M (Preis für die DDR: 12, – M); Bandpreis 180, – M zuzüglich Versandspesen (Preis für die DDR: 120, – M).

Bestellnummer dieses Heftes: 1054/22/3.

AN (EDV) 64914

Die Nahrung

ISSN 0027-769X

Chemie, Biochemie, Mikrobiologie,
Technologie, Ernährung

22. Jahrgang 1978 Heft 3

Akademie für Landwirtschaft in Szczecin, Institut für Technologie der Meeresnahrungsmittel, Abteilung Mikrobiologie der Lebensmittel (Leiter: Prof. Dr. habil. St. ZALESKI, VR Polen)

Empfindlichkeit von Meeresbakterien gegenüber einigen in der fischverarbeitenden Industrie eingesetzten Desinfektionsmitteln. 1. Mitt. Homologe und heterologe Resistenz von *Pseudomonas* und *Moraxella spp.*

St. ZALESKI und I. STOPIKOWSKA

Es wird nachgewiesen, daß Stämme von *Moraxella* spp. gegen die quartäre Ammonium- und Pyridinbasen (QAPB) enthaltenden Desinfektionsmittel Sterinol und Laurosept nur eine schwache Resistenz ausbilden. Bei Stämmen von *Pseudomonas* spp. wird dagegen eine erhebliche homologe und heterologe Resistenz gegen Sterinol und Laurosept beobachtet. Bei 5monatiger Aufbewahrung der resistenten Stämme im QAPB-freien Medium tritt ein teilweiser Resistenzverlust auf. Keiner der untersuchten Meeresbakterienstämme wurde gegen Chloramin T resistent. Die gegen Laurosept und Sterinol resistenten Stämme werden gegen Chloramin T empfindlicher. Obwohl diese Keime keine Chloramin-T-Resistenz ausbilden, werden sie infolge des Kontakts mit subletalen Konzentrationen dieser Verbindung gegen QAPB empfindlicher.

Auch bei einer richtig durchgeführten Desinfektion werden nicht alle Mikroorganismen abgetötet. Im Falle des Einsatzes von quartären Ammonium- und Pyridinbasen (QAPB) vermögen die überlebenden Keime eine Resistenz auszubilden [1—6]; die gebräuchlichen Konzentrationen der Präparate werden dann unwirksam.

In Polen werden zur Zeit 2 Desinfektionsmittel hergestellt, die aktive QAPB enthalten, und zwar Lauryl-dimethyl-benzylammoniumbromid (Handelsname: Sterinol) und Laurylpyridinbromid (Laurosept). Es handelt sich um Kationendetergentien, deshalb ermöglichen sie das Benetzen der Oberfläche und wirken als emulgierender Faktor. Sie verlieren ihre biologische Aktivität bei richtiger Lagerung nicht, sind fast atoxisch für Mensch und Tier und haben ein breites Wirkungsspektrum [7—12]. Die QAPB verdanken ihre bakterizide Wirkung der Fähigkeit, auf die Zellwand einzuwirken; dabei wird die Durchlässigkeit der zytoplasmatischen Zellmembran verändert, was zum Tode der vegetativen Zelle führt [13—14]. Sie wirken ferner zerstörend gegenüber Viren und einigen Pilzen [7, 8, 12]. Der Mechanismus der Einwirkung von QAPB auf Viren ist noch wenig bekannt; man vermutet eine mögliche mechanische Wirkung [7]. Die entkeimende Wirkung von Sterinol gegenüber Pilzen hat TADEUSIAK untersucht [12]; sie hat die abtötende Wirkung dieses Präparats nicht nur auf vegetative Formen, sondern auch auf Sporen einiger Gattungen nachgewiesen.

QAPB verbinden in sich also eine Reihe von sehr günstigen Eigenschaften; ungünstig ist der Verlust bzw. die erhebliche Reduzierung der antibakteriellen Aktivität in Gegenwart von organischen Substanzen wie Seifen und oberflächenaktiven anionischen Verbindungen [8, 9, 11, 15—17].

Jeder Zweig der Lebensmittelindustrie weist eine charakteristische Mikroflora auf. Für die Fischindustrie sind besonders die Meeresbakterien bedeutend, darunter eine Reihe von Fäulnisstämmen der Art *Pseudomonas, Moraxella* u. ä. Die Wirksamkeit von Laurosept gegenüber der Mikroflora der afrikanischen Fische untersuchte KOCHANOWSKI [8] und stellte eine höhere Empfindlichkeit der Bakterien gegen dieses Präparat im Vergleich zu Sulfapol fest; sein Nutzen für die Fischindustrie wird damit positiv eingeschätzt.

Mit unseren Untersuchungen wurde beabsichtigt, die natürliche Empfindlichkeit der Fäulnisstämme von Meeresbakterien gegen Sterinol und Laurosept und als Vergleich gegen Chloramin T zu bestimmen. Gleichzeitig sollte bei diesen Stämmen eine Resistenz gegen QAPB erzeugt werden, um den Unterschied zwischen der Ausgangsempfindlichkeit der Stämme und der Empfindlichkeit der resistenten Stämme festzustellen.

Material und Methoden

Material

Die untersuchten Stämme wurden von der National Collection of Marine Bacterium in Torry Research Station-Aberdeen erhalten:

- *Pseudomonas fluorescens* (Gr. I) NCMB 129 — Ps. 129,
- *Pseudomonas sp.* (Gr. III/IV) NCMB 130 — Ps. 130,
- *Moraxella sp.* NCMB 132 — Mor. 132,
- *Pseudomonas sp.* (Gr. III/IV) NCMB 224 — Ps. 224,
- *Moraxella sp.* NCMB 308 — Mor. 308,
- *Pseudomonas sp.* (Gr. II) NCMB 320 — Ps. 320,
- *Pseudomonas fragi* (Gr. II) NCMB 1353 — Ps. 1353,
- *Pseudomonas putrefaciens* NCMB 1733 — Ps. 1733,
- *Pseudomonas sp.* (Gr. I) NCMB 1792 — Ps. 1792.

Unter den Stämmen von *Pseudomonas spp.* befinden sich die für den Fischverderb aktivsten Gattungen.
Im folgenden werden für die Kennzeichnung der Stämme die angegebenen Abkürzungen verwendet.
Als Nährböden dienten:

- synthetisches Meerwasser (SMW): 23,4 g NaCl; 0,66 g KCl; 3,91 g Na_2SO_4; 0,19 g $NaHCO_3$; 4,96 $MgCl_2$; dest. Wasser zu 1000 ml.
- flüssiger Nährboden (FN): 5,0 g Bacto Peptone; 3,0 g Hefeextrakt; 750 ml SMW; 250 ml dest. Wasser.
- Agarnährboden (AN): 15,0 g Bacto Agar (Difco); 1000 ml FN.
- Agar zur Geldiffusion (AG): 10,0 g Bacto Agar (Difco); 1000 ml FN.

pH-Wert der Nährböden 7,3.
Ausgangsdesinfektionsmittel waren:

- Sterinol, 10%ige wässerige Lösung,
- Laurosept, 25%ige wässerige Lösung,
- Chloramin T, wasserfreies Natriumsalz des N-Chlor-p-toluolsulfamids.

Methoden

Bestimmung der Ausgangsempfindlichkeit mittels Plattenmethode. Die Stämme wurden auf AN, die unterschiedliche Konzentrationen des Desinfektionsmittels enthielten, geimpft; als Ausgangskonzentration galt diejenige Konzentration, bei der kein Wachstum erfolgte.

Resistenzsteigerung gegen ein Desinfektionsmittel. Die bei der jeweils höchsten Konzentration des Desinfektionsmittels gewachsenen Kolonien wurden alle 72 h auf AN mit der gleichen und höheren Konzentrationen überimpft bis zur Stabilisierung der Unempfindlichkeit, d. h. bis zur Grenze der Steigerung der Resistenz. Eine Stabilisierung galt als gegeben, wenn mindestens dreimal keine Empfindlichkeitsänderung zu verzeichnen war. Bei Stämmen, die resistent wurden, stellten wir die Empfindlichkeit gegenüber einem heterologen Desinfektionsmittel fest.

Relative homologe und heterologe Resistenz. Die homologe Resistenz wurde berechnet, indem die Größe der erworbenen Unempfindlichkeit durch ihre Ausgangsresistenz dividiert wurde. Die heterologe Resistenz ist als Kreuzresistenz zu betrachten. Nach der Resistenzausbildung gegenüber einem Desinfektionsmittel wurde die Höhe der Resistenz gegenüber einem anderen Desinfektionsmittel berechnet.

Geldiffusion. Die Empfindlichkeit der sensiblen und resistenten Stämme wurde, wie bei Antibiotika, mittels Loch-Test bestimmt. Es wurden verwendet: 0,3%ige wäßrige Lösungen von Sterinol und Laurosept sowie eine 1%ige wäßrige Lösung von Chloramin T. Bei der Ablesung der Ergebnisse differenzierten wir 2 Zonen: die Zone der völligen Wachstumshemmung (I) und die Zone des selektiven Wachstums (II).

Stabilität der Resistenz. 1. Resistente Stämme wurden 9mal je 72 h auf AN überimpft ohne Zusatz von Desinfektionsmitteln; anschließend wurde ihre Resistenz gegen ein homologes Desinfektionsmittel bestimmt. 2. Resistente Stämme wurden auf AN über 150 Tage bei +4 °C aufbewahrt; in dieser Zeit wurden sie 5mal überimpft. Nach dieser Zeit wurde ihre homologe und heterologe Resistenz festgelegt.

Untersuchungsergebnisse

Die Ausgangsempfindlichkeit der untersuchten Stämme gegen QAPB ist unterschiedlich und schwankt im Bereich von 0,0004% bis 0,08% (Tab. 1). Die höchste Ausgangsempfindlichkeit auf dem Nährboden mit Sterinol und Laurosept wiesen Stämme Mor. 132, Mor 308 und Ps. 224 auf (Abb. 1 und 2). Die niedrigste Empfindlichkeit gegen Sterinol zeigten Ps. 1353, Ps. 1792, Ps. 320 und Ps. 129 und gegen Laurosept Ps. 1353 und Ps. 1792.

Nach Stabilisierung der Empfindlickeit auf der höchsten Stufe wurde nach den Passagen die größte Unempfindlichkeit gegen Sterinol bei Stämmen Ps. 1792 und Ps. 129 sichtbar; sie wuchsen noch bei 2,6%iger Konzentration (Tab. 1). Hinsichtlich Laurosept zeigte Ps. 130 das Wachstum bis zu einer Konzentration von 2% (Abb. 2). Im Falle von Chloramin T kann man nicht von Resistenzbildung sprechen, da ihre Unempfindlichkeit nur von 0,15% auf 0,45% gestiegen ist. Die Steigerung der relativen Resistenz gegenüber Laurosept (Tab. 2) betrug das 3,3fache beim Stamm Mor. 132 und ging bis zum 72,5fachen bei Ps. 129; die übrigen Stämme lagen dazwischen. Eine Ausnahme bildete hier Ps. 130, bei dem diese Resistenz um das 666fache erhöht ist. Bezüglich Sterinol wiesen 4 Stämme eine geringe Resistenzsteigerung auf; bei den übrigen 5 Stämmen erreichte sie mehr als das 100fache (Ps. 1733 3714fach, Pt. 130 1300fach).

Die relative heterologe Resistenz war in der Relation Laurosept — Sterinol und umgekehrt bei Ps. 130 sehr hoch (226—250fach); bei den übrigen Stämmen lag sie zwischen 1,2 und 16,6 (Tab. 3).

Tabelle 1
Homologe und heterologe Empfindlichkeitsänderung und Dauerhaftigkeit der Resistenz von Fäulnismeeresbakterien gegen QAPB (Angaben in %)

Basale QAPB	Meeresbakterienstämme	gegen Sterinol Ausgangsempfindlichkeit	gegen Sterinol Grenze der Resistenzsteigerung	gegen Sterinol nach 180tägiger Lagerung	gegen Laurosept Ausgangsempfindlichkeit	gegen Laurosept Grenze der Resistenzsteigerung	gegen Laurosept nach 180tägiger Lagerung
Sterinol	Ps. 1792	0,015	2,6	0,18	—	0,75	0,015
	Ps. 129	0,015	2,6	0,2	—	0,05	0,05
	Ps. 1353	0,015	1,8	0,16	—	0,75	0,05
	Ps. 1733	0,0007	2,6	0,16	—	0,006	0,015
	Ps. 320	0,01	0,06	0,06	—	0,06	0,05
	Ps. 130	0,001	1,3	0,2	—	0,8	0,125
	Ps. 224	0,0007	0,015	0,01	—	0,004	0,004
	Mor. 132	0,0004	0,0005	0,0005	—	0,0009	0,00175
	Mor. 308	0,0005	0,003	0,002	—	0,005	0,0025
Laurosept	Ps. 1792	—	0,09	0,02	0,06	1,7	0,025
	Ps. 129	—	0,25	0,07	0,025	1,8	0,125
	Ps. 1353	—	0,05	0,01	0,08	1,0	0,025
	Ps. 1733	—	0,00085	0,01	0,003	0,06	0,01
	Ps. 320	—	0,015	0,04	0,025	1,2	0,125
	Ps. 130	—	0,25	0,07	0,003	2,0	0,18
	Ps. 224	—	0,01	0,008	0,0009	0,05	0,0025
	Mor. 132	—	0,0005	0,0004	0,0006	0,002	0,00175
	Mor. 308	—	0,001	0,004	0,0007	0,015	0,0025

Tabelle 2
Gesteigerte relative Resistenz von Meeresbakterienstämmen gegen Laurosept, Sterinol und Chloramin T

Meeresbakterienstämme	Laurosept	Sterinol	Chloramin T
Ps. 130	666,0	1300,0	2,6
Ps. 1353	12,5	120,0	3,0
Ps. 320	48,0	6,0	2,6
Mor. 132	3,3	1,2	3,0
Ps. 129	72,5	173,3	1,6
Ps. 224	55,5	21,4	2,2
Ps. 1733	20,0	3714,0	7,5
Mor. 308	21,4	6,0	1,7
Ps. 1792	28,3	173,3	3,0

In einzelnen Fällen blieb die relative heterologe Resistenz in der Relation Chloramin T — QAPB und umgekehrt unverändert oder verminderte sich. Im allgemeinen ist zu beobachten, daß ein gegen QAPB resistenter Stamm gegenüber Chloramin T empfindlicher wird. Die Stämme, die mit subletaler Chloramin-Konzentration in Kontakt waren, werden gegen QAPB empfindlicher.

Mittels Loch-Test wurde die Empfindlichkeit der resistenten und sensiblen Stämme Ps. 1733, Ps. 224 und Mor. 308 untersucht. Nach Tab. 4 haben alle 3 Stämme bei Gegenwart von QAPB eine deutliche homologe und heterologe Resistenz ausgebildet,

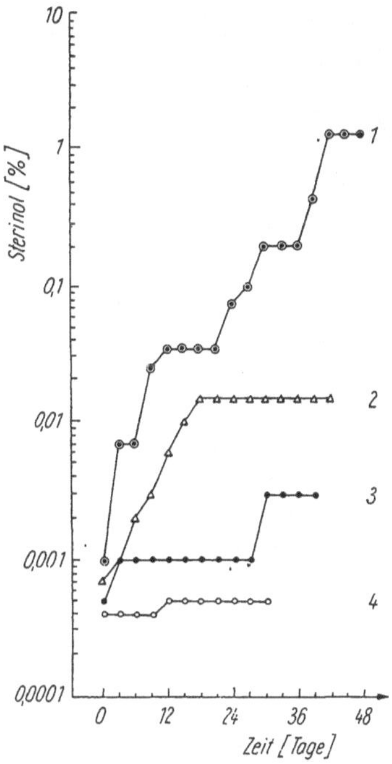

Abb. 1. Resistenzsteigerung von Fäulnismeeresbakterien gegen Sterinol

1 — Ps. 130; 2 — Ps. 224; 3 — Mor. 308; 4 — Mor. 132

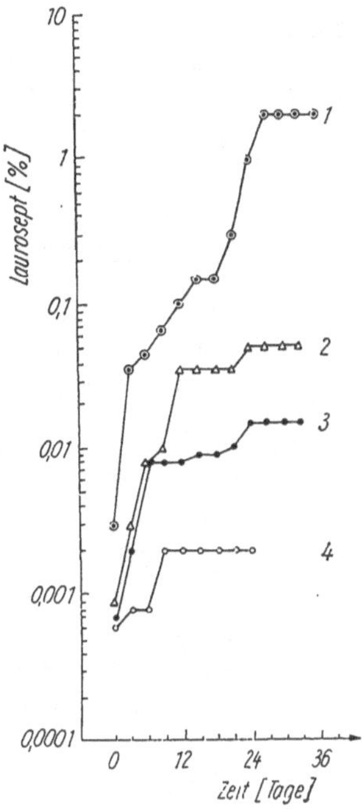

Abb. 2. Resistenzsteigerung von Fäulnismeeresbakterien gegen Laurosept

1 — Ps. 130; 2 — Ps. 224; 3 — Mor. 308; 4 — Mor. 132

Tabelle 3

Gesteigerte relative heterologe Resistenz von Meeresbakterienstämmen gegen Laurosept, Sterinol und Chloramin T

Meeres-bakterien-stämme	Empfindlichkeit gegen Laurosept		Empfindlichkeit gegen Sterinol		Empfindlichkeit gegen Chloramin T	
	gegenüber Sterinol resistenter Stämme	gegenüber Chloramin T resistenter Stämme	gegenüber Laurosept resistenter Stämme	gegenüber Chloramin T resistenter Stämme	gegenüber Laurosept resistenter Stämme	gegenüber Sterinol resistenter Stämme
Ps. 130	266,0	—	250,0	—	—	0,66
Ps. 1353	9,3	0,1	3,3	0,06	1,0	1,0
Ps. 320	2,4	—	1,5	—	0,33	0,13
Mor. 132	1,5	41,0	1,2	20,0	0,66	1,3
Ps. 129	2,2	1,4	16,6	0,66	0,66	0,66
Ps. 224	4,4	—	14,2	—	0,75	0,32
Ps. 1733	2,0	0,2	1,2	—	1,0	1,25
Mor. 308	7,1	—	2,0	—	0,15	0,1
Ps. 1792	12,5	—	6,0	—	1,0	1,3

— = Kein Wachstum bei 0,0001 % und mehr Desinfektionsmittel im Nährboden

Tabelle 4
Einwirkung von Sterinol, Laurosept und Chloramin T auf resistente und sensible Meeresbakterienstämme beim Loch-Test (Angaben in mm)

untersuchte Stämme	Desinfektionsmittel in Löchern des AG					
	Sterinol		Laurosept		Chloramin T	
	Zone I	Zone II	Zone I	Zone II	Zone I	Zone II
Ps. 1733						
A. S.	32,40	37,20	39,60	49,20	23,50	—
S. S.	14,64	36,24	20,40	51,60	20,40	—
L. S.	13,20	32,40	18,00	46,80	22,80	—
C. S.	32,40	—	39,60	—	20,40	—
Ps. 224						
A. S.	27,60	—	34,80	51,60	20,40	—
S. S.	15,60	—	27,60	37,20	20,40	—
L. S.	14,64	—	15,60	18,00	20,40	—
C. S.	29,04	—	37,20	49,20	20,40	—
Mor. 308						
A. S.	34,80	42,00	37,20	46,80	22,80	—
S. S.	25,20	39,60	18,00	27,60	22,80	—
L. S.	25,20	32,40	18,00	25,20	22,80	—
C. S.	34,80	39,60	39,60	46,80	22,80	—

A. S. = Ausgangsstamm
S. S. = gegen Sterinol resistenter Stamm
L. S. = gegen Laurosept resistenter Stamm
C. S. = gegen Chloramin T resistenter Stamm

I = Zone der völligen Wachstumshemmung
II = Zone des selektiven Wachstums
— = keine Zone vorhanden

besonders die Stämme Ps. 1733 und Ps. 224. Gegenüber Chloramin T war die Empfindlichkeit zweier Stämme auf dem gleichen Niveau, und bei Ps. 1733 ist eine geringe Resistenzsteigerung zu verzeichnen. Das Bakterienwachstum in der Zone II im Vergleich zu dem in der Zone I kann auf Dissoziationen des betreffenden Stammes in stärker und weniger stark gegen dieses Desinfektionsmittel empfindliche Bakterienzellen hinweisen. Durch die breitesten Zonen II charakterisiert sich der gegen QAPB resistente Stamm Ps. 1733, bei Ps. 224 sind dagegen seine Zonen unter dem Einfluß von Laurosept begrenzt.

Nach 6facher Überimpfung begann die Resistenz bei den gegen Sterinol resistenten Stämmen Ps. 1733 und Ps. 1353 sowie bei den gegen Laurosept resistenten Stämmen Ps. 1733 und Ps. 320 wieder abzunehmen. Bei den übrigen Stämmen war dies nach 9facher Überimpfung der Fall.

Nach 150tägiger Aufbewahrung bei + 4 °C ist die Resistenz gegen QAPB erheblich gesunken. Wie aus Tab. 1 ersichtlich, sank die Resistenz der Stämme Ps. 1792, Ps. 1353, Ps. 129 und Ps. 1733 gegenüber Sterinol durchschnittlich auf den 13. Teil. Die Empfindlichkeit des Stammes Ps. 1792 gegenüber dem heterologen Desinfektionsmittel erhöhte sich auf das 46fache, bei Ps. 129 und Ps. 224 blieb sie unverändert. Bei den Stämmen Ps. 1733 und Mor. 132 wurde während der Lagerung eine weitere Steigerung der heterologen Resistenz festgestellt, die als sekundäre heterologe Resistenzsteigerung angesehen werden kann. Der Resistenzfaktor betrug bei den erwähnten Stämmen 2,5 und 1,9. Bei den gegen Laurosept resistenten Stämmen verminderte sich die Resistenz schneller, besonders bei Ps. 1792 auf den 64. Teil und bei Ps. 1352 auf den

40. Teil. Die Empfindlichkeit der übrigen Stämme blieb auf hohem Niveau erhalten. Dagegen war die Unempfindlichkeit der gegenüber Laurosept resistenten Stämme gegen Sterinol höher als umgekehrt. Die sekundäre Resistenzsteigerung war wieder für den Stamm Ps. 1733 und diesmal für Mor. 308 und Ps. 320 kennzeichnend.

Diskussion

Bei Kontakt eines Mikroorganismus mit einer subletalen QAPB-Konzentration wird bei einer Reihe von Bakteriengattungen eine Resistenzsteigerung gegen die eingesetzte Verbindung beobachtet [1, 2, 4—6]. Die Resistenzsteigerung ist abhängig von der Gattung des Mikroorganismus; so stieg die Unempfindlichkeit von *Escherichia coli* auf das 43fache, von *Serratia marcescens* auf das 200fache, und bei Staphylokokken blieb sie unverändert [1]. Bei den Passagen von *Pseudomonas aeruginosa* auf Nährböden mit Sterinol erhöhte sich die Resistenz des untersuchten Stammes auf das 100fache und auf Nährböden mit Laurosept auf das 40fache [4].

Wie unsere Untersuchungen gezeigt haben, entwickelte sich bei Meeresbakterienstämmen von *Pseudomonas spp.* eine bei manchen Stämmen sogar starke Steigerung der Resistenz gegen Sterinol und Laurosept. Von 7 untersuchten Stämmen dieser Gattung zeigten 5 eine über 100mal größere Resistenz (*Pseudomonas putrefaciens* 3714fach). Die Resistenzsteigerung gegen Laurosept war bei diesen Stämmen niedriger, und bei einem von ihnen erhöhte sie sich um das 666fache.

Die Wirksamkeit von QAPB ist von der Gattung der Mikroorganismen [1, 2, 4], vom pH-Wert des Milieus [3, 6, 18] und von der Gegenwart organischer Substanzen abhängig [8, 9, 11, 15, 16].

Bei Benutzung der Ausgangsstämme waren die QAPB im Agarnährboden gegenüber den Pseudomonasstämmen schwächer aktiv als gegenüber den Moraxellastämmen. Die Resistenzsteigerung bei Moraxellastämmen erwies sich als geringfügig, Pseudomonasstämme bildeten dagegen eine homologe und heterologe Resistenz auf dem Niveau aus, bei dem die vom Hersteller empfohlenen Arbeitskonzentrationen von QAPB inaktiv wurden. Infolge des Kontaktes mit subletalen Chloramin-T-Konzentrationen werden die Stämme gegenüber Sterinol oder Laurosept empfindlicher, die gegen hohe Konzentrationen von Laurosept oder Sterinol resistenten Stämme werden hingegen gegenüber Chloramin T sensibler.

Summary

St. Zaleski and I. Stopikowska: Sensitivity of marine bacteria to some disinfectants used in the fish processing industry. Part 1. Homological and heterological resistance of *Pseudomonas* and *Moraxella spp.*

It was shown that ability of developing resistance to QAC by *Moraxella spp.* is limited, while marine strains of *Pseudomonas sp.* are able to develop both homological and heterological resistance to Sterinol and Laurosept. Five months storage in medium without QAC caused partial loss of resistance of strains which previously gained resistance to this compound. None of the tested marine bacteria strains was able to get resistance against Chloramina T. Strains with developed resistance to Laurosept and Sterinol became more sensitive to Chloramina T. On the other hand, as a result of contact of the same bacteria with sublethal doses of Chloramina T increase of sensitivity to QAC was observed.

Резюме

С. Залески и И. Стопиковска: Чувствительность морских бактерий к некоторым, используемым в рыбообрабатывающей промышленности дезинфицирунощим средствам. Сообщ. 1. Гомологическая и гетерологическая устойчивость *Pseudomonas* и *Moraxella spp.*

Прпменённый метод исследования показывает, что способность к приобретению устойчивости штаммов *Moraxella spp.* на ЧАПЩ является слабой, однако у морских штаммов *Pseudomonas spp.* наблюдается ярко выраженная гомологическая и гетерологическая устойчивость против стеринола лауросепта. При содержании штаммов с приобетённой устойчивостью в среде без ЧАПЩ в течение 5 месяцев наблюдается частичная её потеря. Ни одного из исследуемых штаммов не приобретел устойчивость против хлорамина Т. Штаммы, устойчивые против лауросепта и стеринола становятся более чувствительными к хлорамину Т. Те же бактерии после соприкосновения с сублетальными дозами хлорамина становятся более чувствительными к ЧАПЩ.

Literatur

[1] CHAPLIN, C. E., Canad. J. Bot. **29**, 373 (1951).
[2] CHAPLIN, C. E., J. Bact. **63**, 453 (1952).
[3] FISCHER, R., u. P. LAROSE, Nature [London] **170**, 715 (1952).
[4] JASZCZUK, E., u. H. KRZYWICKA, Roczn. PZH **24**, 241 (1973).
[5] KIRCHHOFF, H., Arch. Hyg. **146**, 549 (1963).
[6] WASHAM, C. J., W. E. SANDINE u. P. R. ELLIKER, J. Milk Food Technol. **39**, 273 (1976).
[7] CZERWIŃSKA, E., u. R. KOWALIK, Biul. Inform. Inst. Przem. Organ. **3**, 1 (1973).
[8] KOCHANOWSKI. J., u. M. MACIEJOWSKA, Prace MIR. **14 B**, 183 (1967).
[9] KRZYWICKA, H., Postepy Mikrobiol. **10**, 287 (1971).
[10] SZULC, M., A. STEFANIAKOWA, L. KISZCZAK, D. JAWOREK, J. KOSMÓLSKI u. B. STAŃCZAK, Nowości Wet. **3**, 250 (1973).
[11] SZULC, M., A. STEFANIAKOWA u. B. STAŃCZAK, Medycyna Wet. **29**, 410 (1973).
[12] TADEUSIAK, B., Przem. Spoż. **25**, 370 (1971).
[13] BEAN, H. S., J. appl. Bact. **30**, 6 (1967).
[14] HUGO, W. B., u. M. FRIER, Appl. Mikrobiol. **17**, 118 (1969).
[15] CURRAN, H. R., u. F. R. EVANS, J. Dairy Sci. **33**, 1 (1950).
[16] FEAGAN, L. J., u. D. MURNANE, Austral. J. Dairy Technol. **20**, 55 (1965).
[17] SZULC, M., A. STEFANIAKOWA, B. STAŃCZAK, A. BRUNIAK u. J. MAYER, Przem. Spoż. **25**, 243 (1971).
[18] SOIKE, K. F., D. MILLER u. P. R. ELLIKER, J. Dairy Sci. **25**, 764 (1952).

Prof. Dr. habil. St. ZALESKI Akademie für Landwirtschaft, Institut für Technologie der Meeresnahrungsmittel, Kazimierza Królewicza 3, 70—550 Szczecin, VR Polen.

Eingegangen 6. 7. 1977

Die Nahrung	22	3	1978	275–283

Institute of Engineering and Biotechnology of Food
(Director: Prof. Dr. habil J. JAKUBOWSKI), Agrotechnical Academy, Olsztyn, Poland

Use of Glucose-Galactose Concentrates in Beer Production

S. POZNAŃSKI, J. LEMAN, W. BEDNARSKI, W. SZMELICH,
J. KOWALEWSKA, M. CHODKOWSKI and R. WIELICZKO

Three kinds of demineralized and non-demineralized glucose-galaktose concentrates obtained from whey or partially refined lactose, were substituted for barley malt in brewers wort. Demineralized concentrates can be substituted for up to 50% of the malt extract in wort without negatively affecting the technological process of beer production or the quality of the final product. Beer produced with concentrates added showed high quality, flavour and smell, being in most cases quantitatively superior to the control beer. Substitution for the extract by non-demineralized concentrate showed that while a 10% substitution did not negatively affect the quality of beer, increased proportions of 25 and 50 per cent produced a salty taste.

The increasing consumption of beer induces producers to look for other sugar substitutes for malt. ZIEGLER [13] singles out three essential groups of malt substitutes:

1. Non-malted raw starches (barley, maize, rice, millet)
2. Malt products, spitzmalz, malt flakes, green malt
3. Such concentrates as: wort concentrates obtained from barley through an enzymatic method, green malt extract, glucose syrup obtained by an acidic or enzymatic hydrolysis of starch, or even saccharose.

A tendency of use of whey in producing various types of beer has been observed in recent years. HOLSINGER et al. [6] states after ROEDER that partially deproteinated whey, previously boiled at pH 4.5 to 5.5 together with hop cones, can serve as substitute for 3% of the malt. DIETRICH [3] describes the production of a beer substitute by mixing a 5.4 per cent malt wort with 2.5 per cent protein-free whey and fermenting the mixture with *Saccharomyces fragiles* yeast. BRAUNER et al. [1] recommend that whey extract could be added to wort for the production of dark beer, however, it was more difficult to maintain good quality of the beer using this method rather than the traditional technology. The increasing world protein shortage means that, increasingly, all proteins are being utilized in milk processing, leading to protein-free whey, which after further refinement, may be a convenient raw material for the production of beer. This paper presents a description of the characteristics and chemical composition of beer produced by partially substituting sugar concentrates from whey for malt wort.

Materials and methods

Three kinds of malt substitues were used in the form of glucose-galactose concentrates obtained from deproteinated whey. Enzymatic hydrolysis of lactose was effected by means of a β-galactosidase preparate derived from the biomass of *Saccharomyces fragilis* yeast [8]. The activity of the β-galactosidase preparate was from 15 to 18 μmol of glucose per mg of the preparate.

To produce a non-demineralized concentrate, enzymatic hydrolysis of the lactose in whey was carried out in the following matter: pH 6.3–6.4, time 7–8 h, temperature 35–40 °C, adding a 2%

β-galactosidase preparate in relation to the amount of lactose. During the hydrolysis more than 80% of lactose was converted into simple sugar. The hydrolysate was pasteurized at 95 °C, filtered and condensed 8 times at 40—60 °C in a vacuum evaporator. The concentrates obtained had a salty-sweet taste with a noticeable whey aftertaste.

Deproteinated whey was demineralized by employing ion-exchange columns and using a highly acidic cation exchanger (Wofatit KPS) and an anion exchanger (Wofatit SBW). The mean load of the ion-exchanger columns was 200 ml/min/l. The demineralized whey was pasteurized at 75 °C, cooled to 37 °C, brought to pH 6.3—6.4, the β-galactosidase preparate added, the lactose was hydrolyzed and filtration and condensation were carried out as above. Sweet syrups with a pleasant taste and a straw-yellow colour were obtained.

Raw lactose was obtained according to the known technology [7] from defatted and deproteinated whey remaining after the production of cheese or curds. The moist lactose crystals were washed twice with water at 1—2 °C in the proportion 1:1. The purified lactose crystals were dissolved in water at 60 °C, yielding a 4% lactose solution which was cooled to 40 °C and then exposed to enzymatic hydrolysis, filtration and condensation as above. A sweet sugar concentrate completely free of either a salty or whey after-taste was obtained. A detailed procedure of obtaining the described concentrate was published earlier [10].

In the experiments glucose-galactose concentrates were substituted in amounts of 10, 25 and 50%, for corresponding amounts of the extract in wort, the basis being sugar content of the concentrate. The amount of extract in both the control and test wort (wort + concentrate) was limited at 11 g in 100 g. The extractiveness of the malt used was 75%. Beer with glucose-galactose concentrates was produced according to a method described earlier [9].

Bottom-fermenting beer yeasts of the species *Saccharomyces carlsbergensis* were used for fermentation in the proportion of 1 l thick yeast per 100 l of control wort and test wort. The fermentation was carried out in open tubs at 9—9.5 °C. The beer was stored for 20 days at 0—3 °C with a 0.7 atm carbon dioxide overpressure, after which it was filtered, bottled and stored at 10 °C.

In the initial whey concentrates, the content of dry mass, lactose, reducing sugar, total nitrogen and nonprotein nitrogen, mineral salts and ashes were determined [2]. In addition to this in both control wort and test wort, the content of extract, the content of iso-compounds, and titrimetric and

Table 1
The effect of a non-demineralized glucose-galactose concentrate on the mineral salts content at different stages of wort production

Substitution of extract in wort by concentrate [%]	Stage of wort production	Element [mg/100 ml]			
		Na	K	Mg	Ca
10	before malting	10.42	53.20	6.90	2.05
	before filtration of mash	12.10	55.84	7.20	2.51
	to the wort after filtration	16.30	63.00	7.30	2.35
25	before malting	29.80	80.48	7.20	2.25
	before filtration of mash	31.80	85.00	8.20	3.12
	to the wort after filtration	37.46	95.00	7.50	3.41
50	before malting	62.08	131.00	7.80	3.46
	before filtration of mash	66.68	141.00	8.30	4.56
	to the wort after filtration	68.69	148.00	8.70	4.56
	Control wort	0.63	33.60	6.50	1.33

Table 2
Wort with glucose-galactose concentrate added

Type of concentrate	Substitution of extract by concentrate %	Type of determination					
		Extract [g/100 ml]	Colour EBC units	Acidity [ml 1 N NaOH/100 ml]	pH	Iso-compounds [mg/l]	Total nitrogen [mg/100 ml]
Non-demineralized concentrate	10	11.0	18.0—20.5	1.6	5.8	34	99.8
	25	11.0	19.0—22.5	1.6	5.7	32	92.4
	50	11.0	22.0—25.0	1.6	5.7	31	95.9
Control wort	—	10.8	17.5—17.7	1.6	5.7	34	96.8
Demineralized concentrate	10	11.0	14.4—15.0	1.5	5.5	28	84.0
	25	10.8	12.5—13.1	1.2	5.6	24	74.9
	50	11.0	12.5—13.1	1.1	5.5	24	63.0
Control wort	—	11.1	13.8—14.1	1.5	5.8	33	88.9
Concentrate from partially refined lactose	10	10.8	10.5—11.5	1.5	5.6	29	80.8
	25	11.0	9.4—10.0	1.4	5.6	30	80.0
	50	11.9	9.0— 9.8	1.4	5.6	28	71.6
Control wort	—	10.6	10.7—11.5	1.6	5.6	30	81.0

Table 3
Characteristics of test

Type of beer	Substitution of extract by concentrate [%]	Extract apparent [%]	Extract real [%]	Basic wort [%]	Fermentation apparent [%]	Fermentation real [%]
Beer with addition of non-demineralized concentrate	10	2.58	4.13	10.8	75	62
	25	3.04	4.39	10.2	70	56
	50	3.24	4.41	9.4	65	53
Control beer	—	2.40	4.01	10.8	78	63
Beer with addition of concentrate demineralized on ion-exchangers	10	2.86	4.42	11.0	74	59
	25	3.14	4.60	10.9	71	58
	50	3.75	5.08	10.8	65	52
Control beer	—	2.51	4.19	11.4	78	63
Beer with addition of concentrate obtained from partially-refined lactose	10	3.03	4.50	10.8	72	58
	25	3.25	4.74	11.2	71	58
	50	2.86	4.45	11.2	74	60
Control beer	—	2.56	4.08	10.6	76	61

active acidity were determined, in the beer, the content of apparent and real extract, basic wort, apparent and real fermentation, and alcohol [11]. The colour, in EBC units, and commercial durability were determined as well. The quality of the beer was evaluated by group of workers using a 100 point scale [12].

Results and discussion

It is evident from a comparison of the content of dry mass in non-demineralized concentrates (36.4%), concentrates demineralized on ion-exchangers (39.6%), and concentrates obtained from partially-refined lactose (37.2%), against 5.12% in the initial whey that the degree of density of hydrolyzates was more than sevenfold. The content of simple sugars was as follows: 27.4% glucose-galactose and 3.1% lactose (89% of hydrolysis); 34.2% glucose-galactose and 2.81% lactose (92% of hydrolysis) and 32.8% glucose-galactose and 75% lactose (92% of hydrolysis).

While the non-demineralized concentrates contained 3.2% ash, in the demineralized concentrates smaller amounts of mineral substances were found, 0.17 and 0.87% when degree of demineralization was 94.7% and 73%, respectively. Similarly, a decidedly lower content of native elements of whey was observed. Their amount in mg/100 ml of concentrate was as follows:

- non-demineralized concentrate: Na — 535.1; K — 1510.2; Mg — 35.4; Ca — 31.2; Cl — 1072.4;
- concentrate demineralized on ion-exchangers: Na — 32.2; K — 22.8; Mg — 1.71; Ca — 0,56; Cl — 24.6;
- concentrate from partially refined lactose: Na — 11.2; K — 286.0; Mg — 22.0; Ca — 62.0; Cl — 300.1.

The differences in the content of ashes and of the described elements affected the level of titrimetric acidity in the concentrates with the non-demineralized at 24.4 °C, and control beer

Alcohol [%]	Acidity [ml 1 N NaOH/ 100 ml]	pH	Colour in EBC units	Isocompounds [mg/l]	Nitrogenous substances total [mg/100 ml]	Nitrogenous substances coagulable N [mg/100 ml]	Commercial durability [days]
3.38	2.2	4.5	13.0—14.0	24	46.4	2.55	19
2.94	2.2	4.6	14.0—14.5	24	49.0	1.96	9
2.53	2.6	4.8	11.0—12.0	26	57.4	2.31	—
3.53	2.0	4.6	12.8—13.7	22	44.8	1.82	23
3.40	2.4	4.2	10.0—11.0	16	57.4	—	58
3.21	2.0	4.4	9,0—10.0	16	45.8	—	50
2.92	2.1	4.2	9.0—10.0	21	38.5	—	58
3.69	2.1	4.3	9.0—10.0	18	56.7	—	42
3.22	2.0	4.5	7.0—7.5	24	47.6	2.80	42
3.32	1.9	4.5	7.5—8.0	23	52.2	3.17	42
3.49	2.1	4.6	7.0—7.5	28	52.5	2.80	42
3.32	1.8	4.4	7.2—7.5	24	51.4	2.73	42

that demineralized on ion-exchangers 6 °SH, and that obtained from lactose 20.5 °SH. No essential differences were found, however, in active acidity which was pH 5.27, 5.33 and 5.22, respectively.

The content of total nitrogen and non-protein nitrogen expressed in mg/100 ml of concentrate was as follows; non-demineralized 368.3 and 308.2, demineralized on ion-exchangers 366.9 and 331.2, and obtained from lactose 168.2 and 159.3. The concentrate derived from partially-refined lactose contained the most favourable level of those nitrogenous compounds which adversely affect beer quality since the affination (partially-refined) eliminated nitrogenous compounds more effectively than mineral salts.

In comparison to control samples, adding a non-demineralized concentrate to the mash prolonged the time of its conversion into sugar. Although a 10% substitution of the wort extract by this concentrate did not effect the process of mash saccharification a 25% substitution lengthened the saccharification time by an average of 30 min and with a 50% substitution saccharification did not occur within 60 min. Moreover, 25 and 50 substitutions of the concentrate before mashing slightly lengthened the filtration time of wort.

Attempts were also made to substitute a non-demineralized concentrate for part of the wort extract after saccharification of the mash, just before filtration, and directly to the wort after filtration. All 3 methods were of little use because of a considerable increase in the mineral salts content of the test wort (Tab. 1). The most elements were found in the test wort into which the concentrate was added just after filtration, particularly increased amounts of sodium and potassium. The high content of basic elements in the test wort prompted use of demineralized concentrates and concentrates from partially-refined lactose in later experiments.

An analysis of wort in which 3 types of concentrates had been substituted for the malt extract showed that, regardless of the type of concentrate added, the required extract in wort (11 g/100 g $\pm$ 0,4) could be obtained with no difficulty (Table 2).

The colour of wort varied greatly (9.0—25.0 in EBC units) due to differences in the colour of the malt. However, the addition of both demineralized concentrates and those obtained from lactose caused only a slight lightening of the colour of wort, the greater change in the case of the lactosal concentrate. Conversely, adding a non-demineralized concentrate darkened the wort. Wort acidity was decreased slightly with the addition of the concentrate obtained from lactose but increased with the addition of that demineralized on ion-exchangers. No differences in pH were observed between control and test worts.

With the exception of the non-demineralized concentrate, adding concentrates to the wort decreased the total content of nitrogenous compounds in the test worts proportionate to the amount of concentrate added (Table 2).

The amout of apparent extract in the control beer tended to increase with the increased addition of concentrate, while apparent fermentation slightly decreased (Table 3). The alcohol content in all samples of test beer decreased with increasing additions of extract, greater differences being observed in beer with a non-demineralized concentrate, and lesser in beer with the concentrate derived from partially refined lactose. A higher titrimetric acidity was found in the beers than in the worts which produced them, particularly in that with the addition of a non-demineralized concentrate (Tables 2 and 3). Slight differences in active acidity ($\pm$0.1 pH unit) were found in all samples of the test beer. In beer with an addition of non-demineralized concentrate the concentration of hydrogen ions exceeded the acceptable level of the quality standard for Pilsner-type beer, being pH 4.5—4.8 as against 4.4—4.7 pH [5]. In other samples of the test beer pH was up to the quality standard.

The colour intensity in the test beer approximated the control beer, differences between each of the test series resulting from differences in colour of the initial wort (Table 3).

The content of nitrogenous substances (total N and coagulation N) was fully satisfactory with the exception of the beer with a non-demineralized concentrate (Table 3).

The commercial durability of the test beer produced by adding of demineralized concentrates was not only very good but greater than that of the control beer. The beer with concentrates obtained from lactose also showed good durability, identical to that of the control beer, whereas the beer with an addition of a non-demineralized concentrate showed unsatisfactory durability, lower than that of the control beer.

The results of sensory evaluation using a 100 point classification, have been presented in Table 4. The series of samples on beer manufactured with partially-refined lactosal concentrate added received the highest score (80.7—82.8), higher than the control beer which had 77.3 points. The evaluation of taste and smell proved to be especially favourable at 30—30.2 points as against 27.9 points for the control beer, with foamines scoring 9.6—10.0 as against 9.1 points, respectively. Similarly the samples with concentrates demineralized on ion-exchangers were favourably with 76—78 points as against 77.3 for the control beer.

The evaluation of the tests on beer with non-demineralized concentrate added proved unsatisfactory as follows: substituting 10% of extract with concentrate — 76 points; 25% — 70.8 points; 50% — 50.3 points. A salty aftertaste was the main reason for the low quality of beer with a 50% substitution rate, and for this reason the content of basic elements in both test and control beer was determined. The high

Table 4
Mean results of sensory evaluation of beer with an addition of glucose-galactose concentrate to the wort

Type of beer	Substitution of extract by concentrate [%]																				
	10	25	50	10	25	50	10	25	50	10	25	50	10	25	50	10	25	50	10	25	50
	Foamines			Clarity			Colour			Saturation			Bitterness			Flavour			Total points		
Beer with non-demineralized concentrate	8.0	8.7	5.7	9.1	8.2	4.0	4.3	4.0	4.1	8.3	8.2	6.7	18.4	17.7	16.0	27.9	24.0	19.8	76.0	70.8	56.3
Beer with concentrate demineralized on ion-exchangers	10.0	10.0	10.0	8.6	8.6	8.6	4.4	4.4	4.4	8.2	8.4	8.4	17.6	18.4	17.4	27.8	28.8	27.2	76.6	88.0	76.5
Beer with concentrate obtained from partially-refined lactose	10.0	9.6	10.0	9.2	9.1	9.2	5.0	5.0	5.0	9.0	8.5	9.0	18.3	18.3	19.2	30.0	30.2	30.2	81.5	80.7	82.8
Control beer	9.1			9.0			4.6			8.5			10.2			27.9			77.3		

Table 5
Elements present in beer produced with an addition of glucose-galactose concentrates

Type of beer	Substitution of extract by concentrate [%]	Elements [mg/100 ml] Na	K	Mg	Ca
Beer with non-demineralized concentrate	10	23.6	106.5	7.45	12.0
	25	47.8	121.0	9.35	18.4
Beer with concentrate demineralized on ion-exchangers	10	1.65	33.7	5.5	3.2
	25	2.09	37.7	5.8	3.3
	50	2.63	42.7	5.8	3.4
Control beer	—	1.29	36.9	6.1	2.85
Beer with concentrate obtained from partially-refined lactose	10	6.15	52.7	6.33	3.63
	25	9.67	60.3	6.36	5.90
	50	15.80	72.8	6.55	8.65
Control beer	—	1.20	38.1	5.53	2.76

content of mineral salts in beer with non-demineralized concentrates added does not differ from the content of those ingredients in the wort (Tables 1 and 5).

The use of a concentrate demineralized on ion-exchangers causes manifold reductions in the content of mineral salts as compared with the beer produces with an addition of a non-demineralized concentrate. The salts content in this series of test beer kept within the limits found in beer produced from barley malt [11]. The content of the designated elements in the beer with an addition of concentrate derived from partially refined lactose was higher than in the control beer. In particular, a higher content of potassium and calcium was found, with the amount of magnesium only slightly higher. The higher content of salts in the series of beer was not perceptible organoleptically by several workers and beer consumers.

The positive results achieved in this paper show the possibility of employing sugar concentrates from whey in the production of beer. It is possible to show, using Poland as an example, that assigning only 50% of the annual output of whey, i. e. 1.7×10^6 litres, for the production of sugar concentrates, and substituting those for about 25% of the malt extract in beer would yield savings of 35 thousand tons of barley annually. This might enable either an increase in beer production or the use of barley in other branches of food industry.

Zusammenfassung

S. POZNAŃSKI, J. LEMAN, W. BEDNARSKI, W. SZMELICH, J. KOWALEWSKA, M. CHODKOWSKI und R. WIELICZKO: Einsatz von Glucose-Galaktose-Konzentraten in der Bierherstellung

Drei Arten von entsalzten und nichtentsalzten Glucose-Galaktose-Konzentraten aus Molke oder aus teilweise gereinigter Lactose wurden bei der Herstellung von Bierwürze zum Austausch gegen Gerstenmalz eingesetzt. Bis zu 50% des Malzextraktes in Bierwürze können durch entsalzte Konzentrate ohne negative Beeinflussung des technologischen Ablaufs der Bierproduktion und der Qualität des Endproduktes ersetzt werden. Die unter Verwendung solcher Konzentrate hergestellten Biere waren von hoher Qualität, gutem Geruch und Geschmack; sie waren in den meisten Fällen den Vergleichsbieren überlegen. Der Austausch von 10% Malzextrakt durch nichtentsalzte Konzentrate beeinflußte die Bierqualität nicht negativ, aber ein Austausch von 25 oder 50% führte zu einem salzigen Geschmack.

Резюме

С. Позناньски, Я. Леман, В. Беднарски, В. Шмэлих, Я. Ковалевска, М. Ходковски и Р. Величко: Применение галактозо-глюкозовых концентратов в производстве пива

Употреблялись три различных заменителей солода в пивном сусле в виде деминерализованных и недеминерализованных глюкозо-галактозовых концентратов, полученных непосредственно из сыворотки или из частично очищенного сахара. Энзиматичны гидролиз лактозы происходил при помощи энзиматичного препарата β-галактозидазы.

Применение полученных из частично очищённой лактозы и геминерализованных при помощи ионитов концентратов при производстве пива делает возможным заменить до 50% экстракта в пивном сусле без отрицательного влияния на технологический процесс и качество готового продукта.

Пиво полученное с добавкой этих концентратов отличалось хорошими органолептическими свойствами и превышало качество контрольной пробы.

При замене экстракта в пивном сусле недеминерализованным Концентратом показалось, что заменена экстракта в количестве 10% не влияет отрицательно на качество готового пива. При применении более высоких добавок недеминерализованного концентрата (25 и 50%) можно было обнаружить солёный привкус из — за присутствиям минеральных солей.

References

[1] BRUNNER, R., and A. VOGL, Gambrinus **5**, 181 (1944); Chem. Zbl. **115** II, 1128 (1944).
[2] BUDSŁAWSKI, J., Metody analizy żywności. WPLiS, Warszawa 1967.
[3] DIETRICH, K. R., Brauwissenschaft **1949** (2), 26.
[4] DYLKOWSKI, Browarnictwo, WNT, Warszawa 1974.
[5] HLAVAĆEK, F., Piwowarstwo, WNT, Warszawa 1970.
[6] HOLSINGER, N. H., L. P. POSATI and E. B. VILBISS, J. Dairy Science **57**, 849—859 (1974).
[7] OLSON, T. M., Elements of Dairying, The Macmillan Company, New York 1960.
[8] POZNAŃSKI, S., W. BEDNARSKI, J. KOWALEWSKA, M. MIECZKOWSKI and J. LEMAN, Dokumentacja Instytutu Przemysłu Fermentacyjnego w Warszawie 1975.
[9] POZNAŃSKI, S., W. BEDNARSKI, J. KOWALEWSKA, W. DYLKOWSKI and J. JAKUBOWSKI, Patent PRL Nr. 178102 (1975).
[10] POZNAŃSKI, S., M. MIECZKOWSKI, W. BEDNARSKI, J. KOWALEWSKA, J. LEMAN and A. CHRZANOWSKA, Przemysł Spożywczy **31**, 62 (1977).
[11] Praca zbiorowa — Kontrola chemiczna-techniczna produkcji słodu i piwa, WPLiS, Warszawa 1959.
[12] Zarządzenie Wewnętrzne Zjednoczenia Przemysłu Piwowarskiego Nr. 20 z dnia 14-V-1963.
[13] ZIEGLER, G., Brauwelt **109**, 39, 559 (1969).

Prof. Dr. S. POZNAŃSKI, Institute of Engineering and Biotechnology of Food, Agrotechnical Academy, Olsztyn, Poland

Eingegangen 12. 7. 1977

Die Nahrung	22	3	1978	285—289

Institute of Nutrition (Director: Prof. Dr. R. TARJÁN), Budapest, Hungary

The Role of Biogenic Amines in Foods

V. TARJÁN and G. JÁNOSSY

Biologically active amines are normal constituents of many foods for example cheese, plant foods and wines. These low molecular weight organic bases do not represent any hazard to individuals, unless large quantities are ingested or natural mechanism of their catabolism are inhibited.
Investigations were performed concerning the histamine and tyramine content of the Hungarian made cheese, domestic vegetables, fruits and some other foods.
In this paper we should like to draw the attention to the problems of amines from the point of view of food hygiene and food-drug interactions.

Biogenic amines are formed by decarboxylation of amino acids as a consequence of metabolic processes in animals, plants and microorganisms. Biologically active substances — even in relatively small quantities — develop different physiological effects. Chemically they are defined as low molecular weight aliphatic, alicyclic or heterocyclic organic bases. As to the mechanism of effect, biogenic amines are generally either psychoactive or vasoactive. Psychoactive amines act as neural transmitters in the central nervous system (as for example, dopamine, norepirephrine) while vasoactive amines act either directly or indirectly on the vascular system (for example, the pressor effect of tyramine or histamine — being a strong capillary dilator — can produce hypotensive effects.)
Biologically active amines are normal constituents of many foodstuffs, but they usually do not represent any hazard to individuals, unless large quantities are ingested or the natural mechanism for the catabolism of the amines is inhibited for various reasons.

Here are some factors that govern formation of biologically active amines in foods:

1. presence of free amino acids;

2. microorganisms that can decarboxylate the amino acids. According to literature data and to our own investigations some of these microorganisms that are able to produce biogenic amines include: *E. coli*, *Aerobacter*, *Salmonella*, *Shigella*, *Pseudomonas*, *Streptococcus*, *Clostridium*, *Proteus*, *Morganella*, etc.;

3. favourable conditions for the growth of the microorganisms and for the production of decarboxylase enzymes. But from the hygienic point of view these conditions are extremely unfavourable. The determination, that the presence of biogenic amines in foods is the indicator of the unfavourable hygiene, is generally acknowledged.
Numerous studied literature reports emphasize the particular role of biogenic amines in food poisonings of unknown etiology, and that the biogenic amines are such pharmacologically active substances, which have the potential for either pro-

ducing a pharmacological effect, or interacting with different drugs to produce unexpected reactions.

These circumstances stimulated our laboratory to determine the content of biogenic amines (and first of all that of tyramine and histamine) in different foods.

Materials and methods

Different foodstuffs were obtained in groceries and markets. 20 g of the samples were measured. From samples of fruits, vegetables and fishes extractions were made by adding 40 ml of methanol.

The filtrate made of the methanol extract was layed on Whatman 3 paper. 20 g of cheese sample was homogenized with 40 ml physiological salt solution. The homogenate was centrifugated (0 °C, 10000 RPM), then filtered. The filtrate was loaded onto an ionexchange column (Amberlit IRC 50 (H)), previously cleaned by the method of HIRS et al. [6]. The column was several times washed with distilled water, than twice eluated with 15 ml 4 N acetic acid [1]. The eluate was dried up at 40 °C in a rotating evaporator. The evaporated fraction was taken in 1 ml 4 N acetic acid; from this 5—10 µl was dropped on Whatman 3 paper.

In the presence of adequate standards the electrophoresis was carried out in a Laboratory type electrophoretic apparatus (20,3 V/cm and 35 mA) in pyridine — acetic acid buffer (0,01 M pyridine, 0,025 M acetic acid).

After evaporation the spots were developed in ethanol ninhydrin solution and they were evaluated with Chromoscan directly from the paper.

The minimal detectable amount of amines with this method is 1 µg per amine.

Result

Cheese

The largest amount of tyramine was found in hard cheese of long ripening, therefore their consumption is dangerous for the persons sensitive to tyramine. With the decre-

Table 1
Tyramine content of cheese [mg/100 g]

Name of the sample (number of the samples)	Average	End values
Hard Cheese (21)		
Emmentaler (18)	12.87	5.8—36.0
Cheddar (3)	13.0	6.7—21.0
Semihard Cheese (61)		
Edam (11)	2.56	t—10.2*
Balaton (5)	1.46	1.3—3.1
Tenkes (4)	2.17	1.2—5.0
Trappista (12)	2.62	0.8—7.6
Óvári (9)	2.46	t—4.6
Ilmiçi (3)	1.46	0.7—1.9
Lajta (5)	1.32	t—3.1
Göçsej (5)	1.86	0—7.0
Vadász (4)	3.60	1.9—3.9
Köményes (3)	1.93	0.8—2.8
Processed and smoked Cheese (21)	0.90	0—4.7

The samples containing less than 0.2 g/kg of tyramine are marked with O. Owing to the low sample number some data are only informative.

* trace amount

ase of ripening time the tyramine concentration also diminishes. Similar investigations were made in order to learn the tyramine content in Italy [3], in North America [13], in Turkey [10], and in South Africa [9]. Considering the results, the differences can be explained by determination methods of different sensitivity (chromatographic, electrophoretic, fluorometric), our findings of tyramine concentrations give a good completion to literature data (Table 1).

Similar occurrences were noted while investigating fruits and vegetables. It is well known, that various amines are natural constituents of many plants. According to LOVENBERG [11] the amount of amines is increasing during ripening. The amine level of an over-riped fruit comes up to 10—15th that of the original level.

The explanation for the great differences in the extreme values of amine levels shown in Tables 2 and 3 is, that the 128 samples obtained at the markets were not selected according to their ripening grade.

Fruits, vegetables and some other foods

Our results can hardly be compared with the literature data, presenting much less basis in connection with foods of plant origin. Contrary to negative results of LOVEN-

Table 2
Tyramine content of fruits [mg/100 g]

Name of the sample (number of the samples)	Average	End values
Apple (14)	0	
Pear (5)	0	
Grape (16)	69.1	24—140
Plum (6)	0	
Greengage (3)	t*	
Peach (8)	0	
Currant (1)	0	
Water Melon (1)	46.0	

Table 3
Tyramine content of vegetables [mg/100 g]

Name of the sample (number of the samples)	Average	End values
Potato (3)	84	56—130
Paprika (18)	26.6	0—80
Tomato (14)	25.0	0—120
Cabbage (5)	67.0	44—80
Spinach (6)	28.6	0—68
Common Sorrel (2)	0	
Haricot (4)	16.0	t—23
Carrot (10)	11.9	t—36
Turnip (2)	t	
Cauliflower (1)	40.0	
Cucumber (2)	25.0	
Radish (3)	20.0	
Red Beet (4)	16.0	
Kohlrabi (4)	93.0	34—140

BERG [11], we managed to detect tyramine from all the 16 samples of grapes. In the case of other fruits data were either identical or there were no data at all.

In literature the amine concentration of vegetables, like in case of fruits, was determined by sampling tests, but no comprehensive study or estimation was found.

In Table 4 the results of the analysis of different foods are collected.

Table 4
Tyramine content of other foods

Name of the sample (number of the samples)	Average	End values
Fish		
Tuna (57)	57.45 mg/100 g	t–106
Trout (6)	0	
Bream (6)	43.66 mg/100 g	t–80
Wines		
Red Wines (6)	38.80 μg/ml	10–90
White Wines (13)	110.76 μg/ml	70–212
Chicken liver (10)	5.0 mg/100 g	t–34
Sauerkraut (2)	31.0	

Discussion

The objective of this study is to give an overall picture of occurrences of amines in various foods, and also to compare the literature data with our own results.

Amines, that get into the organism are quickly decomposed by deamination. Most of the tissues contain monoamine oxidase (MAO) enzymes. This mitochondrial enzyme catalyzes the decomposition of many vasoactive amines. From 1960, since MAO inhibitors are used as effective antidepressants, the investigation of vasoactive amines became conspicuous.

If the effect of MAO is blocked by MAO inhibitors, tyramine will get into the circulation system and produce hypertensive reaction. The acuteness of the attacks, depending on the consumed quantity of tyramine, changes from the small headache to cerebral haemorrhage. Thus, tyramine is a symphatomimetic amine of indirect action, discharging noradrenalin from adrenergic neurons, producing its pressor effects. In healthy man 20–80 mg of tyramine injected intravenously cause a marked elevation of blood pressure, at the same time, in individuals on MAO inhibitor as little as 6 mg taken orally can cause a rise in blood pressure [7].

Numerous reports of hypertensive crises leading to death and caused by foods, occur in literature.

Therefore, for patients using MAO inhibitor drugs the consumption of some foods might be dangerous (according to GOODMAN et al. [4] in 1970 3.5 million patients used tranylcypromine, one of many similar drugs). Among these foods are cheese, fermented meat products, some vegetables and fruits, some of the ocean fishes, etc.

The aim of this review was, first of all, to present information on tyramine content of most frequently used foods, and thus point out the danger of some foods — not only cheese — on a rather small population of MAO inhibitor users, and last, but not least, to draw the attention and that of clinicians to an important field of research — the food-drug interaction.

Zusammenfassung

V. TARJÁN und G. JÁNOSSY, Die Rolle der biogenen Amine in Lebensmitteln

Biologisch aktive Amine sind als normale Bestandteile vieler Lebensmittel anzusehen, z. B. von Käse, pflanzlichen Lebensmitteln und Weinen. Diese niedrigmolekularen organischen Basen stellen keine Gefahr für den Menschen dar, wenn nicht große Mengen aufgenommen werden oder ihr natürlicher Abbau gehemmt ist.

Es wurden Untersuchungen über den Histamin- und Tyramingehalt von in Ungarn hergestelltem Käse und von landeseigenen Gemüsen und Früchten sowie einigen anderen Lebensmitteln durchgeführt.

Mit der vorliegenden Arbeit soll die Aufmerksamkeit auf die Amin-Problematik hinsichtlich der lebensmittelhygienischen Aspekte und hinsichtlich der Wechselwirkungen zwischen Lebensmittel und Arzneimittel gelenkt werden.

Резюме

В. Тарян и Г. Яноши: Роль биогенных аминов в пищевых продуктах

Биологически активные амины следует рассматривать как нормальные составные части многих пищевых продуктов, как например сыра, растительных продуктов и вин. Эти низкомолекулярные органические основания не представляют собой опасности для человека, если не потребляются большие количества или нарушено их естественное расщепление.

Проводились исследования содержания гистамина и тирамина в продуцируемых в Венгии сырах, в отечественных овощей и фруктов и в некоторых других пищевых продуктах.

Данной работой внимание обращается на проблематику аминов в отношении пищевой гигиены и взаимодействия между пищевыми продуктами и лекарствами.

References

[1] AWAPARA, J., V. E. DAVIS and O. GRAHAM, J. Chromat. **3**, 11—19 (1960).
[2] BLACKWELL, B., Lancet **1965**, 938—940.
[3] CARNOVALE, E. A., Boll. Soc. Ital. Biol. Sper. **45**, 667—71 (1969).
[4] GOODMAN, L. S., and A. GILMAN, The Pharmacological Basis of Therapeutics, p. 180—184, MacMillan New York 1975.
[5] HARTSHORN, E. A., J. Amer. Diet. Ass. **70**, 15—19 (1977).
[6] HIRS, C. H. W., St. MOORE and W. H. STEIN, J. Biol. Chem. **200**, 493—505 (1953).
[7] HORWITZ, D., JAMA **188**, 1108—1110 (1964).
[8] IENISTEA, C., Microbial Safety of Food, p. 327. Acad. Press. London 1973.
[9] KAPLAN, E. R., Analyst **99**, 565—569 (1974).
[10] KAYAALP, S. O., Tox. Appl. Pharmacol. **16**, 495—460 (1970).
[11] LOVENBERG, W., Toxicants occurring naturally in Foods, p. 170—180, Natl. Acad. Sci., Washington 1973.
[12] RICE, S. L., R. R. EITENMILLER and P. E. KOEHLER, J. Milk Food Technol. **39**, 353—358 (1976).
[13] SEN, N. P., J. Food Sci. **34**, 22—26 (1969).
[14] STAHL, E., Thin layer Chromatography, Springer-Verlag 1969.
[15] VOIGT, M. N., R. R. EITENMILLER, P. E. KOEHLER and M. K. HAMDY, J. Milk Food Technol. **37**, 377—379 (1974).
[16] VOIGT, M. N., and R. R. EITENMILLER, J. Food Protection **40**, 241—245 (1975).

Dr. Veronika TARJÁN und Gizella JÁNOSSY, Institute of Nutrition, Budapest IX, Gyáli-út 3/a, Ungarische VR

Eingegangen 9. 8. 1977

Die Nahrung	22	3	1978	291–297

Abteilung Qualität der Pflanzenprodukte des Instituts für Genetik und Züchtung, Forschungsinstitute für Pflanzenproduktion, Prag, ČSSR

Einfluß der Düngung auf den Eiweißgehalt und auf die Aminosäurenzusammensetzung von Winterweizen in ernährungswissenschaftlich-ökonomischer Hinsicht

J. PRUGAR

Ergebnisse von Düngungsversuchen mit organisch-mineralischer Düngung bei Winterweizen wurden durch Berechnung der Selbstkosten für die Produktion einer Gewichtseinheit der Eiweißstoffe und der essentiellen Aminosäuren in ernährungswissenschaftlich-ökonomischer Hinsicht ausgewertet.

Die Kosten je 1 kg Eiweißstoffe sanken mit steigender Mineraldüngung. Die markantesten Unterschiede traten bei der Variante ohne organische Düngemittel auf; ähnlich verhielt sich auch der Kornertrag.

Die Selbstkosten je 1 kg essentieller Aminosäuren waren in einigen Fällen bei der Kombination Mineral II (max. 160 kg N/ha) höher als die Kosten bei der Kombination Mineral I (max. 120 kg N/ha), da ihr Gehalt im Korn sank. Dies gilt vor allem für die organisch mit Stroh + N gedüngte Variante. Die geringsten Aufwände waren bei der organisch ungedüngten Variante mit höherer Mineraldüngung erforderlich.

Die in der vorhergehenden Arbeit [1] beschriebenen Versuchsergebnisse an Winterweizen wurden ökonomisch ausgewertet, und zwar auf Grund der Berechnung von Selbstkosten, die für die Erzeugung je einer Gewichtseinheit der nutritiv wichtigen Komponenten Eiweißstoffe und essentielle Aminosäuren notwendig sind. Diese bei Düngungsversuchen bisher ungewöhnliche Betrachtungsweise bietet einen neuen Einblick in die Problematik der Pflanzenernährung und der gesamten Weizenanbautechnik. Sie deutet an, daß erst eine komplexe quantitative und qualitative Einschätzung die richtige Antwort geben kann, ob eine bestimmte Maßnahme vom Standpunkt der Produktion jener Komponenten vorteilhaft ist, die für den tatsächlichen Ernährungswert des Weizenkorns für Menschen und Haustiere ausschlaggebend sind.

Methodik

Die Versuchsbedingungen wurden in der vorhergehenden Arbeit [1] beschrieben. In dieser Arbeit wurden die bei gesteigerter Mineraldüngung in zwei Düngungsniveaus gewonnenen Ergebnisse über den Gehalt an Eiweißstoffen sowie an einigen essentiellen und nicht essentiellen Aminosäuren diskutiert. Die Düngung spiegelte sich natürlich auch in unterschiedlichen Selbstkosten für die produzierte Menge der untersuchten Stoffe in den einzelnen Varianten und Kombinationen wider.

Eine höhere Kornproduktion hat zwar eine Steigerung derjenigen Kostenposten zur Folge, die unmittelbar mit der Ernte und der mit der nach der Ernte zu verarbeitenden größeren produzierten Menge je 1 ha zusammenhängen, führt aber gleichzeitig zu einer Senkung der Selbstkosten je Einheit des Produkts.

Die einzelnen Varianten und Kombinationen der Düngung wurden mit Hilfe der Kennzahl „Selbstkosten" für die Produktion von 1 kg Eiweiß und der einzelnen Aminosäuren bewertet. Als Grundlage wurde die Variante ohne Düngung genommen. Es wurde ein Modell mit Kostenposten zusammengestellt, die nach den Normativen je 1 ha berechnet wurden. Die Arbeits- und Materialaufwände wurden in bezug auf den Kornertrag erwogen. Das Modell wurde bei den einzelnen Kombinationen durch die Kosten für die verwendeten Mineraldünger und für die mit der Düngung verbundene Arbeit ergänzt. Mit Rücksicht auf die Nachwirkung der Düngemittel vom Vorjahr wurde zu der verfolgten Getreideart ein Drittel der Kosten für die Kalidüngung und die Hälfte der Kosten für die Phosphordüngung miteinberechnet. Der Wert der Wirtschaftsdünger und die Kosten für die mit ihrer Ausbringung verbundene Arbeit wurden mit Rücksicht auf die vorausgesetzte Wirkung der organischen Dünger auf die Folgefrucht in halber Höhe in die Kosten einbezogen. Bei allen beobachteten Varianten und Kombinationen wurden aus der Summe aller Kostenposten die Gesamtselbstkosten je 1 ha ermittelt.

Bei der eigentlichen Kalkulation, d. h. bei der Bestimmung der Selbstkosten je Einheit des Hauptprodukts, gingen wir so vor, daß wir die einzelnen Aminosäuren schrittweise als Hauptprodukt betrachteten und die Selbstkosten für die Erzeugung der Aminosäuren nach der Formel

$$\text{Selbstkosten für Aminosäuren [Kčs/kg]} = \frac{\text{Gesamtselbstkosten [Kčs/ha]}}{\text{Aminosäurenproduktion [kg/ha]}}$$

berechneten.

Zur Ermittlung der ökonomisch vorteilhaftesten Kombination wurden die Selbstkosten je Einheit der Aminosäuren prozentual mit der weder organisch noch mineralisch gedüngten Kontrolle verglichen.

Ergebnisse und Diskussion

Die in der Tab. 1 aufgeführten Ergebnisse zeigen Unterschiede in den Eiweißerträgen je Flächeneinheit, die durch gesteigerte Mineraldüngung verursacht wurden. Ausgeprägte Unterschiede werden bei der Variante ohne organische Dünger und bei der mit alleiniger Strohdüngung beobachtet. Bei der Variante Stroh + N sind die Unterschiede geringer, da bereits mit dem Stroh bei allen Kombinationen 60 kg Stickstoff pro ha zugeführt werden, so daß der weitere mit dem Mineraldünger gelieferte Stickstoff nur eine weniger markante Wirkung aufweist. Ein ausgeprägt steigender Lysinertrag zeigt sich nur bei der organisch ungedüngten Variante durch Einwirkung der zunehmenden Mineraldüngung (Tab. 1). Bei den Varianten Stroh und Stroh + N ist zwischen den Kombinationen Mineral I und II im Mittel der beiden Jahre praktisch kein Unterschied zu erkennen. Dies entspricht den für die Mittelwerte des Kornertrags und des Lysingehalts in der Korntrockensubstanz gewonnenen Ergebnissen [1]:
Der Kornertrag stieg geringfügig, während der Lysingehalt bei der Kombination Mineral II bereits niedriger war als bei Mineral I. Da der Eiweißertrag (Tab. 1) dabei auch noch bei der Kombination Mineral II stieg, bedeutet dies, daß der Zuwachs an Proteinstoffen vor allem durch Erhöhung der an Lysin armen Eiweißfraktionen verursacht wurde.

Ähnliche Tendenzen kann man auch bei den Mittelwerten der weiteren in Tab. 1 aufgeführten Aminosäuren beobachten. Wenn die einzelnen Versuchsjahre separat beurteilt werden, so ist sichtbar, daß die angeführten Beziehungen im Jahr 1970 ausgeprägter gelten, während sie im nachfolgenden Jahr nicht so deutlich hervortreten. Dies steht offensichtlich damit im Zusammenhang, daß 1971 der Eiweißgehalt auch bei der Kombination Mineral II im Vergleich zu Mineral I weiter anstieg, während er im Vorjahr praktisch gleich blieb.

Tabelle 1
Ertrag an Eiweißstoffen und einigen Aminosäuren [kg/ha]

Variante		Organ. O			Stroh			Stroh + N		
Kombination		Mineral O	Mineral I	Mineral II	Mineral O	Mineral I	Mineral II	Mineral O	Mineral I	Mineral II
Eiweißstoffe	1970	370,8	558,3	622,7	455,2	585,1	654,8	461,5	590,2	608,1
	1971	406,0	615,0	659,1	372,6	591,4	669,5	568,6	633,6	695,5
	Mittel	388,4	586,7	640,9	413,9	588,3	662,2	515,1	611,9	651,8
Lysin	1970	6,80	11,47	16,16	9,59	13,26	14,20	10,99	14,89	12,60
	1971	10,98	15,80	16,83	10,07	16,15	15,97	12,73	15,94	18,01
	Mittel	8,89	13,64	16,50	9,83	14,71	15,09	11,86	15,42	15,31
Threonin	1970	6,30	10,67	14,95	9,38	14,11	13,99	10,42	13,11	11,64
	1971	9,99	13,65	17,74	8,56	12,28	14,57	11,96	15,28	15,99
Valin	1970	11,02	20,25	25,53	16,93	24,44	24,37	17,55	23,35	21,71
	1971	15,64	24,50	27,28	13,14	17,44	23,59	20,31	25,91	25,17
Isoleucin	1970	8,53	14,72	21,69	13,71	19,13	18,28	13,23	18,27	17,00
	1971	13,27	23,15	22,10	10,52	15,20	17,36	16,14	22,13	20,60
Leucin	1970	16,23	27,91	37,24	25,45	35,02	34,49	24,57	33,58	31,70
	1971	22,98	39,85	41,73	20,15	27,93	33,01	25,71	33,27	38,25
Phenyl-alanin	1970	9,87	15,48	25,01	16,54	22,99	22,87	15,48	22,17	20,27
	1971	13,17	21,15	26,52	13,46	15,90	21,73	17,98	23,30	24,81
Prolin	1970	21,71	41,70	55,51	36,19	49,34	56,24	32,96	47,46	49,57
	1971	33,85	51,80	57,33	30,53	38,82	47,95	41,65	49,26	61,09
Glutamin-säure	1970	63,61	116,05	177,55	101,71	144,16	146,68	101,79	137,09	154,26
	1971	82,74	150,25	153,45	89,91	118,29	154,45	102,54	146,09	160,47

Bei den nicht essentiellen Aminosäuren Glutaminsäure und Prolin ist die Korrelation zwischen der Düngergabe und dem Ertrag immer positiv.

Die Selbstkostenbewertung je 1 ha wird in Abb. 1 gezeigt. Die Aufwände steigen mit den gesteigerten Düngemittelgaben. Die höchsten Selbstkosten je 1 ha wurden bei der Kombination Stroh + N und Mineral II aufgewendet, sie betrugen 132% im Vergleich mit der ungedüngten Kontrolle (100%).

Die Erhöhung der Hektarkornerträge durch Einwirkung des in Mineraldünger gelieferten Stickstoffs kam am stärksten bei der organisch ungedüngten Variante zum Ausdruck. Sowohl in den einzelnen Versuchsjahren als auch bei den berechneten Mittelwerten wurden die niedrigsten Kosten je Einheit des Produktes bei den Kombinationen dieser Variante mit Mineraldüngung I und II vermerkt, wo im Mittel um 39,6 bzw. 45,5% höhere Kornerträge und um 51,1 bzw. 65,0% höhere Eiweißerträge im Vergleich zur Kontrolle erreicht wurden.

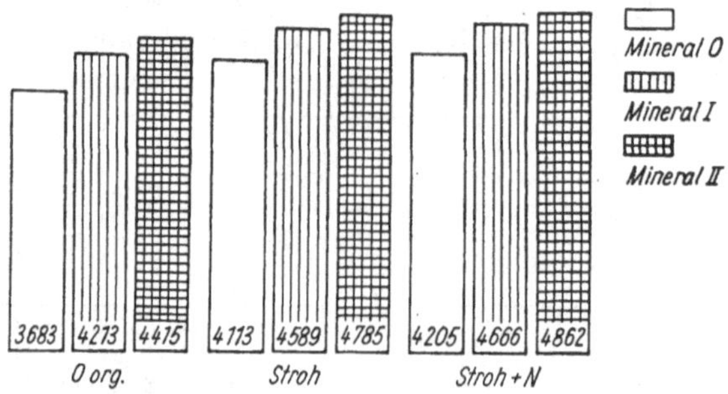

Abb. 1. Selbstkosten der Weizenerzeugung [Kčs/ha]

Tab. 2 veranschaulicht die Selbstkosten für die Produktion von 1 kg Eiweißstoffen. Insgesamt kann festgestellt werden, daß die Kosten bei allen drei Varianten mit gesteigerter Mineraldüngung sinken, d. h. daß Mineraldüngung unter den gegebenen Versuchsbedingungen in den Kombinationen I und II für die Produktion der Eiweißstoffe vorteilhaft ist. Am deutlichsten ist dieser Effekt bei den Varianten ohne organischen Dünger bzw. mit Stroh, während bei der Variante Stroh + N, bei der sich die Mineraldüngung nicht mehr so ausgeprägt im Kornertrag widerspiegelte, die Unterschiede geringer waren.

Die niedrigsten Selbstkosten je 1 kg Eiweißstoffe wurden in beiden Versuchsjahren bei der organisch ungedüngten Kombination Mineral II erhalten; sie lagen um 28,7% (1970) bzw. um 26,2% (1971) niedriger als bei der Kontrolle. Bei der Kombination mit Stroh und Mineral II, bei der im Mittel beider Jahre der höchste Eiweißertrag von 662,2 kg/ha erreicht wurde, liegt die Kostenreduzierung bei 22,7%; bei der aufwendigsten Kombination mit Stroh + N und Mineral II beträgt sie 21,1% bei einem mittleren Eiweißertrag von 651,8 kg/ha.

Die Selbstkosten je 1 kg der einzelnen Aminosäuren (Tab. 2) deuten an, daß sich bei der Variante Stroh + N die oben diskutierte [1] Senkung ihres Gehaltes bei der mit Mineral II gedüngten Kombination im Vergleich zu Mineral I geltend machte. Die bei der Kombination Mineral II für 1 kg essentieller Aminosäuren aufgewendeten Selbstkosten überschreiten häufig die Kosten bei der Kombination I.

Tabelle 2

Selbstkosten für 1 kg Eiweißstoffe und einige Aminosäuren [% zur Kontrolle]

Variante		Organ. O			Stroh			Stroh + N		
Kombination		Mineral O	Mineral I	Mineral II	Mineral O	Mineral I	Mineral II	Mineral O	Mineral I	Mineral II
Eiweißstoffe	1970	100	75,9	71,3	91,2	79,0	73,6	91,5	79,6	80,4
	1971	100	75,6	73,8	124,5	93,7	81,2	81,6	81,2	77,3
Lysin	1970	100	67,8	50,4	79,4	63,9	62,2	70,5	57,8	71,2
	1971	100	79,6	78,2	121,5	84,7	89,4	98,7	87,3	80,5
Threonin	1970	100	67,5	50,5	75,2	55,6	58,5	68,9	60,9	71,4
	1971	100	83,8	67,5	130,1	101,4	89,1	95,6	82,9	82,5
Valin	1970	100	62,2	51,8	72,9	56,2	58,7	71,6	59,8	67,0
	1971	100	73,1	68,7	132,6	111,8	86,2	88,1	76,5	82,1
Isoleucin	1970	100	66,2	47,2	69,7	55,6	60,6	73,5	59,1	66,2
	1971	100	65,6	72,0	140,6	108,8	99,4	94,1	76,0	85,1
Leucin	1970	100	66,5	52,3	71,4	57,8	61,1	75,3	61,2	67,6
	1971	100	66,0	66,0	127,1	102,6	90,5	102,3	87,6	79,3
Phenylalanin	1970	100	72,9	47,3	66,8	53,5	56,1	72,7	56,4	64,3
	1971	100	71,3	59,3	109,0	103,2	78,8	83,8	71,7	70,1

Die niedrigsten Kosten je 1 kg Aminosäuren wurden 1970 bei der organisch ungedüngten Variante mit den Kombinationen Mineral I und II erhalten, bei der die Kostensenkung im Vergleich zur Kontrolle im Mittel aller beobachteten essentiellen Aminosäuren 50,1% beträgt. Bei der Kombination Stroh + N und Mineral II (mit den höchsten Kosten je ha) sanken die Kosten je 1 kg essentieller Aminosäuren beim Vergleich zur Kontrollvariante im Mittel um 32,1% und bei der Variante nur mit Stroh um 40,5%.

1971 wurden Höchsterträge der beobachteten essentiellen Aminosäuren bei der Kombination ohne organische Düngung und Mineral II erhalten; sie lagen im Mittel um 76,9% höher als die Kontrolle. Bei der aufwendigsten Kombination Stroh + N und Mineral II wurden im Mittel um 66,0% höhere Erträge erreicht. Nur im Fall von Lysin wurde die höchste Menge bei der Kombination Stroh + N und Mineral II und von Isoleucin bei der organisch ungedüngten Kombination mit Mineral II produziert.

Im Hinblick auf die erreichten Erträge der essentiellen Aminosäuren und die auf die einzelnen Varianten und Kombinationen aufgewendeten Gesamtkosten erwies sich 1971 wieder die organisch ungedüngte Kombination mit Mineral II als am effektivsten.

Die Strohapplikation wirkte sich auch bei Kombination mit N im Jahre 1971 nicht so günstig aus wie im Vorjahr, und bei der Kombination Stroh + Mineral O trat in diesem Jahr sogar eine Erhöhung der Selbstkosten im Mittel aller beobachteten Aminosäuren um 26,8% ein. Dieser Einfluß äußerte sich auch noch bei der Kombination Stroh + Mineral I, bei der sich – mit Ausnahme von Lysin – die Kosten je Einheit der sonstigen beobachteten Aminosäuren im Mittel um 4,6% erhöhten. Der Grund hierfür ist dem niedrigeren Gehalt an essentiellen Aminosäuren im Korn in diesem Jahr zuzuschreiben, offensichtlich als Folge der abklingenden Luzerneeinwirkung aus den Jahren 1967–68. Der zugeführte Stickstoff wurde vor allem für die Ertragsbildung sowie für die Bildung von biologisch unterwertigen Eiweißfraktionen verwertet. Im Verlauf der Kornbildung stand Stickstoff nicht mehr in einer für die Eiweißsynthese genügenden Menge zur Verfügung.

Die Mineraldüngerapplikation bei den organisch ungedüngten und mit Stroh gedüngten Varianten führte in der Regel mit zunehmender Mineraldüngung zur Kostensenkung je Einheit des Produkts, während sich bei der Variante Stroh + N die Düngung mit Mineral I effektiver in den Kosten zeigte. Bei Zufuhr von Mineral II haben sich die Kosten je Einheit im Vergleich mit Mineral I nicht so deutlich reduziert; bei einigen Aminosäuren sind sie sogar höher.

Meinem Mitarbeiter Herrn Dipl.-Ing. HUGO ROB danke ich für die technische Hilfe bei der Bearbeitung dieser Publikation.

Summary

J. PRUGAR: The effect of fertilization on the protein content and amino-acid composition of winter wheat from the viewpoints of the science of nutrition and of economics

The results from experiments on the organo-mineral fertilization of winter wheat were evaluated from the viewpoints of the science of nutrition and of economics by calculating the prime cost for producing one unit of weight of proteins and essential amino acids.

The prime cost for 1 kg of proteins decreased with the increase of mineral fertilization. The most marked differences were observed with the variant „without organic manure". The crop yield showed a similar behaviour.

In certain cases, the prime cost per kg of essential amino acids was higher with the combination Mineral II (max. 160 kg N/ha) than with the combination Mineral I (max. 120 kg N/ha), because of reduced content in the grain. This applies above all to the variant ,,straw + N". Expenditure was lowest in the variant ,,no organic manure and high mineral fertilizer".

Резюме

Й. Пругар: Влияние удобрения на содержание белка и аминокислотный состав озимой пшеницы с точки зрения питания и экономики

Результаты экспериментов по удобрению озимой пшеницы органически-минеральным удобрением анализировались с помощью расчета себестоимости продукции одной весовой единицы белковых веществ и незаменимых аминокислот с точки зрения питания и экономики.

С тоимость 1 кг белковых веществ снизилась с увеличением минерального удобрения. Наиболее значительные различия наблюдаются при использовании варианта без органического удобрения; подобно изменился и урожайность зерна.

Себестоимость на 1 кг незаменимых аминокислот в некоторых случаях была выше при комбинации минерала II 160 кг N/га) чем стоймость при использовании комбинации минерала I (120 кг N/га), так как их содержание в зерне снижалось. Это относится особенно к варианту, где органическое удобрение производили с помощью соломы + N. Наименьшие затраты наблюдались при неорганическом варианте с высоким содержанием минерального удобрения.

Literatur

[1] Prugar, J., Nahrung **22**, 163 (1978).

Doz. Dipl.-Ing. J. Prugar, CSc., Forschungsinstitute für Pflanzenproduktion, Institut für Genetik und Züchtung, 161 06 Praha 6 — Ruzyně, ČSSR

Eingegangen 29. 8. 1977

Die Nahrung	22	3	1978	299—307

Abteilung Qualität der Pflanzenprodukte des Instituts für Genetik und Züchtung, Forschungsinstitute für Pflanzenproduktion, Prag, ČSSR

Einfluß der Düngung auf den Thiamin- und Riboflavingehalt von Winterweizen

J. PRUGAR

In Feldversuchen (1970 und 1971) mit je zwei Mineraldüngungsgaben (max. 120 bzw. 160 kg N/ha) auf organisch ungedüngten, mit Stroh gedüngten bzw. mit Stroh + N gedüngten Varianten wurden der Thiamin- und Riboflavingehalt von Winterweizen untersucht. Die Düngung wirkte sich auf den Gehalt der beiden Vitamine im Vergleich mit der ungedüngten Kontrolle günstig aus. Bei Thiamin wurden bessere Ergebnisse bei Kombinationen mit einer niedrigeren Stickstoffgabe erreicht, während bei Kombinationen mit Gesamtzufuhr von 160 kg N/ha in Form von Mineraldüngemitteln bereits eine schwache Senkung vermerkt wurde. Bei Riboflavin waren die Unterschiede weniger ausgeprägt.
Bei höheren Stickstoffgaben steigt der Gehalt an Rohprotein schneller an als der Gehalt der beiden Vitamine. Da sich hierbei vor allem der Gehalt der Prolaminfraktion erhöht, wird gefolgert, daß eine engere Korrelation des Gehaltes an Thiamin und an Riboflavin mit den höherwertigen Albumin- und Globulinfraktionen besteht als mit dem Gesamtgehalt der N-Stoffe.
Es wurden die Erträge der beiden Vitamine je Flächeneinheit sowie die für die Produktion von 1 g notwendigen Selbstkosten berechnet. Bei Thiamin erwies sich die intensivere Düngung in beiden Versuchsjahren als weniger ökonomisch, bei Riboflavin war dies nur 1971 der Fall.

Die vorliegende Arbeit bringt weitere Forschungsergebnisse in bezug auf den nutritiven Wert des Korns von Winterweizen, der in mehrjährigen Feldversuchen der Forschungsinstitute für Pflanzenproduktion Prag-Ruzyně in den Jahren 1969—1971 bei Applikation verschiedener Gaben organischer und mineralischer Düngemittel angebaut wurde. Die Studie knüpft damit an vorhergehende Publikationen [23, 24] an. Gegenstand der vorliegenden Arbeit ist der Gehalt des Weizens an zwei wichtigen Vitaminen der B-Gruppe, dem Thiamin und Riboflavin.

Bisherige Untersuchungen über den Gehalt an Vitaminen betreffen vor allem den Einfluß der Sorten und die im Verlauf der Mühlenverarbeitung entstandenen Verluste. Durch derartige Analysen wurden die meisten Angaben über den Thiamin- und Riboflavingehalt im Korn (Tab. 1 und 2) erhalten.

JAHN-DEESBACH u. a. [12] führen auch einige ältere Arbeiten an, bei denen die Einflüsse des Standorts, vor allem der Bodenart, und der Niederschläge während der Vegetationsperiode sowie in geringerem Ausmaß auch die Wirkung verschiedener Düngung auf den Thiamingehalt untersucht wurden. Die gewonnenen Ergebnisse deuten an, daß unter weniger günstigen Bedingungen für die Kornentwicklung, z. B. in trockenen Jahrgängen, der Vitamingehalt in der Regel steigt, da durch die geringere Stärkeanhäufung im Korn kein sogen. „Verdünnungseffekt" auftritt.

Was die Düngungseinflüsse betrifft, stimmen europäische Autoren [7, 8, 21, 27, 28] mit amerikanischen überein [2, 5, 31], wonach eine erhöhte Stickstoffdüngung den Thiamin- und in geringerem Ausmaß auch den Riboflavingehalt im Weizenkorn günstig beeinflußt und in der Regel mit dem Eiweißgehalt parallel verläuft.

Die wichtigste Arbeit der letzten Jahre über den Einfluß der Stickstoffernährung auf den Vitamin-B_1-Gehalt im Weizenkorn publizierten die bereits erwähnten Autoren JAHN-DEESBACH u. a. [12].

Tabelle 1

Thiamingehalt im Weizenkorn nach verschiedenen Autoren

Autoren	Jahr der Veröffentlichung	Thiamingehalt [mg/100 g]
KRETOVIČ [17]	1954	0,37–0,61
PRUGAR [22]	1960	0,35–0,42 (i. T.)
FRAGNER u. a. [9]	1961	0,33–0,55
MOWSZOWICZ [19]	1963	0,43–0,67
WATT u. a. [34]	1963	0,43–0,57
SINIC u. a. [30]	1965	0,35–0,50
PRUGAR u. a. [26]	1970	0,36–0,63
KALINA [15]	1971	0,22–0,41
MEREDITH u. a. [18]	1971	0,53–0,62 (i. T.)
ADRIAN u. a. [1]	1972	0,48–0,57
JAHN-DEESBACH u. a [12]	1972	0,33–0,60
TOEPFER u. a. [33]	1972	0,54–0,67 (i. T.)
KALINA [16]	1973	0,31–0,45
ŠAŠKINA u. a. [32]	1973	0,53
Eigene Ergebnisse	1978	0,35–0,56 (i. T.)

Anmerkung: Falls nicht anders angegeben, beziehen sich die Werte auf einen Gehalt an Trockensubstanz von 85–91%
i. T. = in Trockensubstanz

Tabelle 2

Riboflavingehalt im Weizenkorn nach verschiedenen Autoren

Autoren	Jahr der Veröffentlichung	Riboflavingehalt [mg/100 g]
DEVJATNIN [6]	1948	0,08–0,09
CALHOUN u. a. [4]	1958	0,14–0,20
JERMAKOV [14]	1958	0,06–0,11
GASSMANN u. a. [10]	1959	0,12–0,14
SCHWEIGART u. a. [29]	1959	0,23
MOWSZOWICZ [19]	1963	0,09
SINIC u. a. [30]	1965	0,12–0,22
JANICKI u. a. [13]	1967	0,08–0,20
SHUPHAN u. a. [28]	1968	0,10–0,18 (bez. auf einen Gehalt an Trockens. von Ø 81–90%)
BARTLOVÁ [3]	1970	0,07–0,22
CHRZANOWSKA [11]	1970	0,08
KALINA [15]	1971	0,07–0,12
MEREDITH u. a. [18]	1971	0,11–0,14 (i. T.)
ADRIAN u. a. [1]	1972	0,085
TOEPFER u. a. [33]	1972	0,11–0,12 (i. T.)
KALINA [16]	1973	0,06–0,12
NOVÁKOVÁ u. a. [20]	1973	0,12–0,21
Eigene Ergebnisse	1978	0,08–0,15 (i. T.)

Anmerkung: Falls nicht anders angegeben, beziehen sich die Werte auf einen Gehalt an Trockensubstanz von 85–91%
i. T. = in Trockensubstanz

Sie untersuchten den Thiamingehalt von Proben aus acht Winterweizen- und sechs Sommerweizensorten aus einem 1968 angelegten Düngungsversuch, und zwar bei Varianten, in denen Stickstoff in zunehmenden Gaben in späten Vegetationsphasen zugeführt wurde. Eine signifikante Erhöhung des Thiamingehalts infolge der Stickstoffzusatzdüngung wurde bei der Mehrzahl der 14 untersuchten Sorten ermittelt, wobei wesentliche sortenbedingte Unterschiede festzustellen waren. Diese Erscheinung ist der unterschiedlichen Sortenreaktivität auf die Zusatzdüngung zuzuschreiben, wo in einigen Fällen die Ertragssteigerung die Vitaminbildung übertrifft, was wieder zu dem bereits erwähnten „Verdünnungseffekt" führt.

Sortenbedingte Einflüsse wurden von uns nicht verfolgt. Das Ziel unserer Versuche war es, den Einfluß verschiedener organischer und mineralischer Düngung auf die Thiamin- und Riboflavinbildung zu untersuchen und auf diese Weise an einem Modell die Möglichkeiten zu prüfen, die die Weizenernährung auf die Gehalte dieser wichtigen Kennwerte des nutritiven Wertes des Korns bietet.

Methodik

Eine ausführliche Charakteristik der Versuchsstellen, die Beschreibung der Witterungsbedingungen in den beobachteten Jahren sowie Angaben über die Art der Düngung bei den einzelnen Varianten und Kombinationen wurden in der vorangehenden Arbeit [23] angeführt. In dieser Arbeit sind auch Daten über die erreichten Kornerträge angegeben.

Es wurden folgende analytische Methoden verwendet:

Thiamin wurde fluorometrisch mit Hilfe der Thiochrommethode bestimmt, Riboflavin ähnlich mit Hilfe der Lumiflavinmethode. Beide Verfahren wurden ausführlich in unseren früheren Arbeiten [10, 25, 26] beschrieben.

Die in den Tabellen für die einzelnen Jahrgänge aufgeführten Werte sind Mittel von zwei parallel durchgeführten Analysen. Die Durchschnittswerte aus beiden Jahren sind demnach aus vier analytischen Ergebnissen berechnet worden.

Ergebnisse und Diskussion

Aus Tab. 3 kann abgeleitet werden, daß sich die Mineraldüngung auf den Thiamingehalt günstig auswirkte, die niedrigsten Werte wurden in der Regel bei der ungedüngten Variante Mineral O beobachtet. Eine zunehmende positive Tendenz zwischen gesteigerten Düngungsgaben und Thiamingehalt kann bei der organisch ungedüngten Variante und im Jahr 1970 auch bei der Variante mit Stroh beobachtet werden. Bei der Variante Stroh + N bewirkt die weitere Zufuhr von Mineralstoffen (vor allem Stickstoff) nicht mehr einen Zuwachs des Gehaltes an Vitamin B_1, es wurde im Gegenteil in beiden Jahren eine schwache Verminderung bei der Kombination Mineral II im Vergleich zu Mineral I erhalten.

Es zeigte sich daher, daß für die Thiaminsynthese bei den erzielten Kornerträgen, der gegebenen Sorte und den äußeren Bedingungen bei der Variante Stroh + 60 kg N/ha bereits die weitere Gabe von 60 kg N/ha in Form von Mineraldünger zum Erreichen des Maximalgehaltes an Thiamin im Korn genügte. Die Zufuhr von 100 kg N/ha als Mineraldünger führte bei der Kombination Mineral II (insgesamt 160 kg N/ha) über-

Tabelle 3
Thiamingehalt im Korn [mg/100 g TM]

Variante	Organ. O			Stroh			Stroh + N		
Kombination	Mineral O	Mineral I	Mineral II	Mineral O	Mineral I	Mineral II	Mineral O	Mineral I	Mineral II
1970	0,41	0,44	0,45	0,38	0,42	0,48	0,42	0,52	0,50
1971	0,45	0,45	0,53	0,42	0,51	0,50	0,50	0,56	0,52
Mittel	0,43	0,44	0,49	0,40	0,47	0,49	0,46	0,54	0,51

Tabelle 4
Riboflavingehalt im Korn [mg/100 g TM]

Variante	Organ. O			Stroh			Stroh + N		
Kombination	Mineral O	Mineral I	Mineral II	Mineral O	Mineral I	Mineral II	Mineral O	Mineral I	Mineral II
1970	0,119	0,120	0,136	0,113	0,126	0,122	0,115	0,119	0,120
1971	0,083	0,083	0,099	0,099	0,088	0,093	0,099	0,099	0,105
Mittel	0,101	0,102	0,118	0,106	0,107	0,108	0,107	0,109	0,113

Tabelle 5
Thiaminertrag [g/ha]

Variante	Organ. O			Stroh			Stroh + N		
Kombination	Mineral O	Mineral I	Mineral II	Mineral O	Mineral I	Mineral II	Mineral O	Mineral I	Mineral II
1970	12,01	17,64	19,44	13,60	17,85	20,59	14,74	22,00	21,80
1971	15,87	22,49	26,87	14,49	25,35	25,75	24,30	28,62	26,99
Mittel	13,94	20,07	23,16	14,05	21,60	23,17	19,52	25,31	24,40

wiegend zur Erhöhung des Kornertrages und nur in geringerem Ausmaß zur Thiaminbildung.

Bei Riboflavin sind die Unterschiede zwischen den Varianten und Kombinationen geringer; aus Tab. 4 kann jedoch eine positive Tendenz zum schwachen Anstieg des Gehaltes an Vitamin B_2 mit den höheren Gaben der Mineralernährung entnommen werden. Die Senkung bei der Kombination Mineral II im Vergleich mit Mineral I, die bei der Variante Stroh + N bei Thiamin beobachtet wurde, trat im Falle von Riboflavin nicht ein.

Interessant ist der Vergleich des Gehaltes der beiden Vitamine in bezug auf den Jahrgang: während bei Thiamin im Jahr 1971 ein höherer Gehalt beobachtet wurde (im Mittel aller Varianten und Kombinationen 0,49 mg/100 g im Vergleich mit 0,45 mg/100 g im Jahr 1970) wurden im Gegenteil bei Riboflavin wesentlich höhere Werte im Jahr 1970 ermittelt (0,121 mg/100 g im Vergleich zu 0,094 mg/100 g im Jahr 1971).

Es ist daher wahrscheinlich, daß optimale Bedingungen für die Bildung und Anhäufung im Korn bei beiden Vitaminen nicht gleich sind. Die Bedingungen im Jahr 1970 waren für Riboflavin, diejenigen von 1971 für Thiamin günstiger. Solche Zusammenhänge sind in weiteren Versuchen zu überprüfen.

Tab. 5 und 6 veranschaulichen die Erträge der beiden Vitamine auf einer Flächeneinheit.

Im Vergleich zu der mineralisch ungedüngten Kontrolle bestehen bei den beiden gedüngten Kombinationen bei allen drei Varianten ausgeprägte Zunahmen. Der Unterschied zwischen den Kombinationen Mineral I und Mineral II ist jedoch nur bei Riboflavin bei der Variante ohne organische Düngung signifikant. Bei der Variante mit alleinigem Stroh wurde eine größere Differenz nur bei Thiamin im Jahr 1970 beobachtet; bei der Variante Stroh + N tritt bei der Düngung mit Mineral II bereits eine Senkung ein (im Falle von Thiamin in beiden Jahren, bei Riboflavin nur 1971).

In den Tab. 7 und 8 sind die für die Produktion von 1 g Vitaminen bei verschiedener Düngung aufgewendeten Selbstkosten veranschaulicht.

Es zeigte sich, daß eine Düngung, die gleichzeitig den Ertrag und den Vitamingehalt steigert, sich günstig durch Senkung der Produktionskosten auswirkt. Bei Thiamin hat sich bei der Variante Stroh + N die Kombination Mineral II ökonomisch bereits weniger günstig ausgewirkt, und die Kosten stiegen im Vergleich zur Kombination Mineral I wieder an (im Jahr 1971 auch bei der Variante mit alleinigem Stroh); bei Riboflavin trat diese Erscheinung 1970 bei Stroh und 1971 bei Stroh + N auf.

Erkenntnisse über Beziehungen zwischen dem Gehalt an N-Stoffen und Thiamin im Weizenkorn

Jahn-Deesbach u. a. haben in ihrer genannten Arbeit [12] positive Korrelationen zwischen dem Thiamingehalt und dem Rohproteingehalt im Korn festgestellt. Auf diese Weise wurden die Ergebnisse einiger früherer Arbeiten [2, 21, 31] bestätigt. Die Verfasser machen jedoch gleichzeitig darauf aufmerksam, daß diese positiven Beziehungen nicht für jeden einzelnen Fall gelten müssen, da sie offensichtlich von sortenbedingten Eigenschaften stark abhängig sind.

Unsere in den vorangehenden Arbeiten [23, 24] sowie in dieser Studie angeführten Ergebnisse ergänzen weitgehend die Beobachtungen der oben genannten Autoren. Vor

Tabelle 6
Riboflavinertrag [g/ha]

Variante	Organ. 0			Stroh			Stroh + N		
Kombination	Mineral 0	Mineral I	Mineral II	Mineral 0	Mineral I	Mineral II	Mineral 0	Mineral I	Mineral II
1970	3,46	4,21	6,39	4,65	6,04	5,23	3,83	5,03	5,67
1971	2,93	4,15	5,02	3,42	4,37	4,79	4,81	5,89	5,45
Mittel	3,20	4,18	5,71	4,04	5,21	5,01	4,32	5,46	5,56

Tabelle 7
Selbstkosten für 1 g Thiamin [Kčs]

Variante	Organ. 0			Stroh			Stroh + N		
Kombination	Mineral 0	Mineral I	Mineral II	Mineral 0	Mineral I	Mineral II	Mineral 0	Mineral I	Mineral II
1970	306,0	238,1	226,6	302,6	256,6	231,9	284,1	211,6	222,5
1971	232,5	187,8	164,6	283,7	181,4	186,2	173,7	163,4	180,5
Mittel	269,3	213,0	195,6	293,2	219,0	209,1	228,9	187,5	201,5

Tabelle 8
Selbstkosten für 1 g Riboflavin [Kčs]

Variante	Organ. 0			Stroh			Stroh + N		
Kombination	Mineral 0	Mineral I	Mineral II	Mineral 0	Mineral I	Mineral II	Mineral 0	Mineral I	Mineral II
1970	1062,1	997,6	689,5	884,9	758,3	912,0	1093,5	925,4	855,6
1971	1259,0	1018,1	881,1	1202,0	1052,2	1001,0	877,5	794,1	893,9
Mittel	1160,6	1007,9	785,3	1043,5	905,3	956,5	985,5	859,8	874,8

allem wurde die positive Beziehung zwischen dem Eiweißgehalt und dem Thiamingehalt im Korn bestätigt. Sie kann auch für Riboflavin gelten, wo allerdings in unserem Falle bei der Sorte Mironovska die Veränderungen des Gehaltes an Vitamin B_2 durch die Einwirkung der Düngung nur gering waren; die Tendenz war jedoch offensichtlich. Angaben für weitere Sorten und abweichende ökologische Bedingungen sind bisher nicht vorhanden, jedoch werden sie 1979 zur Verfügung stehen, und zwar nach Auswertung der derzeitig durchgeführten Feldernährungsversuche mit dieser Sorte an mehreren Stellen in Böhmen und Mähren.

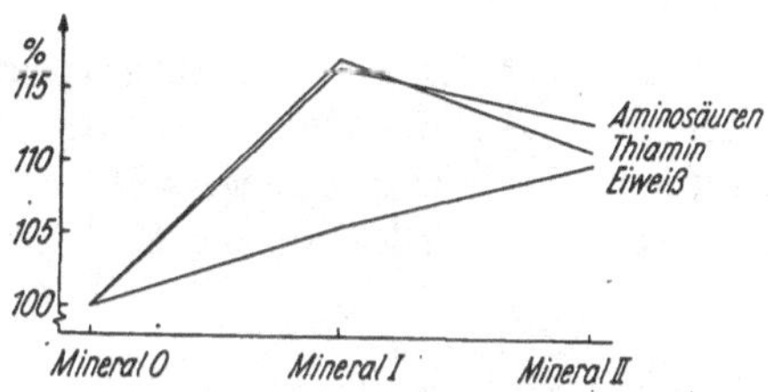

Abb. 1. Vergleich der Thiamin-, Eiweiß- und Aminosäurengehalte bei verschiedener Düngung

Die Stickstoffdüngung wirkt sich daher in der Regel sowohl durch Anstieg des Eiweißgehaltes als auch der beiden Vitamine der B-Gruppe aus. Bei höheren Gaben von Stickstoff kommt es jedoch in einigen Fällen (in Abhängigkeit von der Sorte sowie vom Gesamtkomplex der Vegetationsbedingungen) zur Reduzierung des Thiamingehaltes, während der Eiweißgehalt weiter steigt. Durch detaillierte elektrophoretische Analyse der Eiweißstoffe und Bestimmung ihrer Aminosäurenzusammensetzung haben wir festgestellt, daß die prozentuale Erhöhung der Eiweißstoffe vor allem zu Lasten derjenigen Fraktionen geht, die arm an essentiellen Aminosäuren sind [23]. Bei der Variante Stroh + N und der Kombination Mineral II, wo die gesamte in Mineralform zugeführte Stickstoffmenge 160 kg/ha betrug, trat meist bei den verfolgten essentiellen Aminosäuren, ebenso wie bei Thiamin, eine Senkung des Gehaltes im Vergleich mit der niedrigeren Mineral I-Kombination (120 g N/ha) ein, d. h. es lag ein „Verdünnungseffekt" vor. Aus diesen Tatsachen kann die Hypothese abgeleitet werden, daß zwischen dem Thiamingehalt und den essentiellen Aminosäuren eine engere Korrelation besteht als zwischen dem Gehalt an diesem Vitamin und Rohprotein. Die in Abb. 1 aufgeführten Mittelwerte der beiden beobachteten Jahrgänge bestätigen diese Vermutung. Die Korrelationen waren 1970 besser als 1971, in dem die Ergebnisse stärker schwankten und der Gehalt an einigen essentiellen Aminosäuren auch bei der höheren Stickstoffgabe (Mineral II) weiter anstieg.

Eine aus diesen Beobachtungen folgende praktische Schlußfogerung ist, daß die agroökologischen Faktoren, die den nutritiven Wert des Weizenkorns hinsichtlich seiner Aminosäurenzusammensetzung günstig beeinflussen, gleichzeitig auch eine positive Wirkung auf die Bildung von Vitamin B_1 und umgekehrt ausüben.

Es kann vorausgesetzt werden, daß in den Fällen, wo Jahn-Deesbach u. a. [12] bei einigen verfolgten Sorten nur einen geringfügigen Zuwachs an Thiamingehalt bei höheren späten Stickstoffgaben von 60 bzw. 100 kg/ha beobachteten, während der Rohproteingehalt bis zu 40% zunahm, vor allem Prolaminfraktionen erhöht wurden, die hinsichtlich des nutritiven Wertes minderwertig sind. Die Bestimmung der Aminosäurenzusammensetzung hätte wahrscheinlich gezeigt, daß der Gehalt an essentiellen Aminosäuren gleich blieb bzw. langsam stieg, ähnlich wie der Thiamingehalt.

Die von den genannten Autoren gestellte Frage, ob der hohe Rohproteingehalt eine Voraussetzung für einen hohen Thiamingehalt darstellt, kann daher negativ beantwortet werden. Die Thiaminsynthese verläuft bei genügender Stickstoffzufuhr parallel mit der Synthese der Eiweißstoffe mit ausgeglichener Bildung aller Fraktionen. Sobald jedoch die Stickstoffzufuhr eine bestimmte Grenze überschreitet, wird der Stickstoff vor allem für die Synthese von Prolamin-Eiweißfraktionen verwertet, während die Bildung nutritiv hochwertiger Eiweißbestandteile sowie des Thiamins rückläufig wird.

Selbstverständlich kann bei diesen Erscheinungen eine spezifische sortenbedingte Reaktivität erwartet werden, die auch die oben genannten Verfasser hervorgehoben haben, sowie evt. Unterschiede in bezug auf verschiedene äußere Bedingungen. Weitere Untersuchungen werden zweifellos in dieser Hinsicht interessante Beziehungen klären.

Meinem Mitarbeiter, Herrn Dipl.-Ing. HUGO ROB, danke ich für die technische Hilfe bei der Bearbeitung dieser Publikation.

Summary

J. PRUGAR: The effect of fertilization on the thiamine and riboflavin contents of winter wheat

The author studied in field trials (1970 and 1971) the effect of two amounts of mineral fertilizer (max. 120 and 160 kg N/ha, respectively) in combination with the variants "no organic manure", "straw" and "straw + N" on the thiamine and riboflavin contents of winter wheat. As compared to the control ("no organic manure"), the fertilization had a beneficial effect on the contents of both vitamins. With regard to thiamine, better results were achieved by combinations with the lower amount of fertilizer nitrogen, whereas combinations with a total amount of 160 kg N/ha in the form of mineral fertilizers already produced a slight decrease. These differences were less marked with riboflavin.

If higher amounts of nitrogen were applied, the content of raw protein increased more rapidly than that of both vitamins. Since in this case the prolamin content is increased above all, it is concluded that the thiamine and riboflavin contents are more closely correlated with the albumin and globulin fractions than with the total nitrogenous substance content.

The yields of both vitamins per unit of area and the prime cost for the production of 1 gramme were calculated. The more intense fertilization was less economic for thiamin in both years of trial; for riboflavin, only in 1971.

Резюме

И. Пругар: Влияние удобрения на содержание тиамина и рибофлавина у озимой пшеницы

В двух экспериментах в полевых условиях в 1970 и 1971 годах исследовалось содержание тиамина и рибофлавина озимой пшеницы после удобрения двумя вариантами минерального удобрения (120 или 160 кг *N*/га) без органического удобрения, с удобрением соломой или соломой + *N*.

Удобрение оказало благоприятное действие на содержание обоих витаминов по сравнению с неудобренным контролем. В отношении тиамина более хорошие результаты наблюдались при комбинации с более низкой дозой азота, в то время как комбинации с общей дачей 160 кг *N*/га в форме минерального удобрения приводили к легкому снижении. В отношении рибофлавина различия менее выражены.

При даче более высокой дозировки азота содержание натурального белка возрастает быстрее чем содержание обоих витаминов. Поскольку увеличивается в первую очередь содержание проламина, делается вывод, что существует более тесная связь между содержанием тиамина и рибофлавина с одной стороны и ценными альбуминовыми и глобулиновыми фракциями чем с общим содержанием N-веществ.

Расчитывалась неоходимая себестоимость для продукции I г витамина и продукция обоих витаминов на единицу площади. Для тиамина интенсивное удобрение в двух исследованных годах оказалось малоэффективным, в отношении рибофлавина это имело место только для 1971 года.

Literatur

[1] ADRIAN, J., u. L. PETIT, Tec. Molitoria 23, 5—27 (1972).
[2] BAINS, G. S., Cereal Chem. 30, 139—145 [1953).
[3] BARTLOVÁ, D., Wiss. Bericht, VÚMPP Praha (1970).
[4] CALHOUN, W. K., W. G. BECHTEL, u. W. G. BRADLEY, Cereal chemistry 35, 350—359 (1958).
[5] CONNER, R. T., u. G. J. STRAUB, Cereal Chem. 18, 671—677 (1941).
[6] DEVJATNIN, V. A., Vitaminy. Piščepromizdat, Moskva (1948).
[7] DÖRING, H., Nahrung 12, 1159—1187 (1960).
[8] DÖRING, H., Deutsche Gärtner-Post 13, 3 (1961).
[9] FRAGNER, J., u. a., Vitaminy, jejich chemie a biochemie. Verlag ČSAV, Praha (1961).
[10] GASSMANN, B., u. H. PLESSING, Z. Lebensmittel-Untersuch. u. -Forsch. 109, 134—145 (1959).
[11] CHRZANOWSKA, H., Biuletyn CLTPPZ Warszawa 14, 62—75 (1970).
[12] JAHN-DEESBACH, W., u. H. MAY, Z. Acker-Pflanzenb. 135, 1—18 (1972).
[13] JANICKI, J. SOBKOWSKA u. J. CHELKOWSKI, Wiss. Bericht WSR, Poznań (1967).
[14] JERMAKOV, A. I., Biochimija kul'turnych rastenij. Tom. I. Sel'chozgiz, Moskvá-Leningrad (1958).
[15] KALINA, J., Wiss. Bericht VÚMPP Praha (1971).
[16] KALINA, J., Wiss. Bericht VÚMPP Praha (1973).
[17] KRETOVIČ, V. L., Zaklady biochemie rostlin. Verlag ČSAV (1954).
[18] MEREDITH, P., u. R. W. CAWLEY, Food Technol. in N. Z. 6, 22—23 (1971).
[19] MOWSZOWICZ, J., Systematyczny przegląd gatunków roślin zawierających witamine C i inne. LTN (1963).
[20] NOVÁKOVÁ, E., u. J. PRUGAR, Rostlinna výroba 19, 533—544 (1973).
[21] PFÜTZER, G., C. PFAFF u. H. ROTH, Landw. Forschung 4, 105—114 (1952).
[22] PRUGAR, J., Rostlinná výroba 6, 115—120 (1960).
[23] PRUGAR, J., Nahrung 22, 163 (1978).
[24] PRUGAR, J., Nahrung 22, 291 (1978).
[25] PRUGAR, J., u. J. VESELÁ, Getreide Mehl 19, 94—95 (1969).
[26) PRUGAR, J., J. VESELÁ, u. E. NOVÁKOVÁ, Rostlinná výroba 16, 219—232 (1970).
[27] SCHARRER, K., u. R. PREISSNER, Z. Pflanzenernährung, Düng., Bodenkunde 67, 166—179 (1954).
[28] SCHUPHAN, W., M. KLING u. G. OVERBECK, Qualitas Plantarum Mater. vegetabiles 15, 177—214 (1968).
[29] SCHWEIGART, H. A., u. G. REHNER, Vitalstoffe-Zivilisationskrankheiten 4, 25—28 (1959).
[30] SINIC, I., u. V. CANIC, Hrana Ishrana 6, 355 (1965).
[31] SPENCER, E., u. M. W. GALGAN, Canad. J. Res. F 27, 450—456 (1949).
[32] ŠAŠKINA, Z. N., u. V. I. ZAJCEV, Izvestija VUZ — Pišč. Technol. 4, 37—38 (1973).
[33] TOEPFER, E. W., M. M. POLANSKY, J. F. EHEART, H. T. SLOVER, E. R. MORRIS, F. N. HEPBURN u. F. W. QUAKENBUSH, Cereal Chem. 49, 173—186 (1972).
[34] WATT, B. K., u. A. L. MERRILL, Composition of Foods. Agricultural Handbook 8., U.S. Dep. of Agric., Washington (1963).

Doz. Dipl.-Ing. JAROSLAV PRUGAR, CSc., Výzkumné ústavy rostlinné výroby, 161 06 Praha 6 — Ruzyně, ČSSR

Eingegangen 29. 8. 1977

Die Nahrung	22	3	1978	309–313

Institut für Ernährung, Sofia, VR Bulgarien

Einfluß einer reduzierten Ernährung und körperlichen Belastung auf die Leberlysosomen. Morphologische und biochemische Untersuchungen

L. Krustev, T. Taschev, A. Pokrovskij, W. Tuteljan, I. Apostolov, L. Krawtschenko und A. Popov

Es werden Gruppen von 15 Ratten (I – freie Ernährung, II – freie Ernährung und körperliche Belastung, III – um 40% reduzierte Ernährung, IV – reduzierte Ernährung und körperliche Belastung) nach 20 bzw. 140 Tagen untersucht. Elektronenmikroskopisch werden die größten Veränderungen in Gruppe III festgestellt; hier liegt ein Überschuß an Autophagolysosomen vor. Die biochemischen Untersuchungen zeigen, daß die reduzierte Ernährung (Gruppe III) auch von einer erheblichen Zunahme der Aktivität der meisten Lysosomenenzyme in der Leber begleitet ist.

Eine auftretende Autophagie zeigt, daß diese entweder physiologisch oder Zeichen eines beginnenden pathologischen Prozesses ist.

Eine Reihe von Untersuchungen zeigt die entscheidende Rolle der Lysosomen als Orte der intrazellulären Verdauung in der Leber beim totalen Fasten [1, 4, 7]. Dabei wird eine neue und besonders wichtige, nämlich die rekonstruktive Funktion dieser Gruppe von Zellorganellen postuliert [5].

Ziel der vorliegenden Arbeit ist die Untersuchung der Teilnahme der Lysosomen an den in der Leber bei reduzierter Ernährung ohne körperliche Belastung sowie unter einer speziellen körperlichen Belastung sich entwickelnden Prozessen.

Material und Methoden

Es wurden 120 männliche weiße Ratten (Wistar, Ausgangsalter 5 Monate, Körpergewicht 220 bis 300 g) untersucht. Die Tiere wurden in individuellen Käfigen gehalten und in 2 Reihen zu je 60 Tieren aufgeteilt. Bei der ersten Reihe dauerte der Versuch 20 Tage, bei der zweiten 140 Tage. In beiden Reihen wurden 4 Gruppen zu je 15 Tieren wie folgt gebildet: Gruppe Ia (20 Tage) und Gruppe I (140 Tage) – freie Ernährung; Gruppe IIa (20 Tage) und Gruppe II (140 Tage) – freie Ernährung und körperliche Belastung; Gruppe IIIa und Gruppe III – reduzierte Ernährung; Gruppe IV – reduzierte Ernährung und körperliche Belastung.

Die freie Ernährung wurde mit Standardfutter (Preßlinge) durchgeführt [2]. Die durchschnittlichen 24std. Werte des aufgenommenen Futters bei freier Ernährung sind: für 4monatige Ratten 24,32 g; für 5monatige Ratten 25,16 g; für 7monatige Ratten 27,33 g; für 8monatige Ratten 22,90 g.

Bei der reduzierten Ernährung wurden 15,00 g Preßlinge/24 h verabfolgt. Das sind gegenüber den frei gefütterten Tieren 60,9% für 4monatige Ratten; 59,7% für 5monatige Ratten; 67,2% für 7monatige Ratten und 64,6% für 8monatige Ratten. Alle Tiere bekamen Wasser ad libitum. Die körperliche Belastung war tägliches Schwimmen bis zur Erschöpfung. Während der ersten 10 Tage variierte die Dauer des Schwimmens zwischen 10 und 15 min, am 20. Tag um 30 min, am 30. Tag um 40 min, am 60. Tag um 60 min, und am 140. Tag lag sie über 75 min.

Ein Stück Leber wurde nach den klassischen histologischen und elektronenmikroskopischen Methoden untersucht. In dem mit Triton-x-100 behandelten Leberhomogenat und in der überstehenden Flüssigkeit (100000 g × 30 min) wurde der Gehalt an Eiweiß nach LOWRY u. a. [3] und an 10 Enzymen der Lysosomen bestimmt: saure Ribonuclease, saure Desoxyribonuclease, β-Glucuronidase, β-Glucosidase, α- und β-Galactosidasen, Arylsulfatase A und B, β-Acetylglucosaminidase, saure Phosphatase und Kathepsin. Die Enzymaktivitäten wurden spektrophotometrisch [6] bestimmt. Die nicht sedimentierte Enzym-Aktivität wurde in Prozent der Gesamtaktivität ausgedrückt.

Ergebnisse

Elektronenmikroskopisch wurde in der Gruppe Ia (Kontrollgruppe) der GOLGI-Appatat dilatiert, außerdem wurden im Zytoplasma einzeln liegende Fett-Tröpfchen mit einem Durchmesser von 2—4 μm beobachtet. Bei der Gruppe IIa (freie Ernährung mit körperlicher Belastung) wurden primäre Lysosomen nicht nur peribiliär, sondern auch im Zytoplasma verstreut gefunden. Bei den Tieren mit reduzierter Ernährung und bei denen mit reduzierter Ernährung und körperlicher Belastung (Gruppen IIIa und IIa) erschienen außer primären auch sekundäre Lysosomen vom Typ der Autophagolysosomen (AFLS).

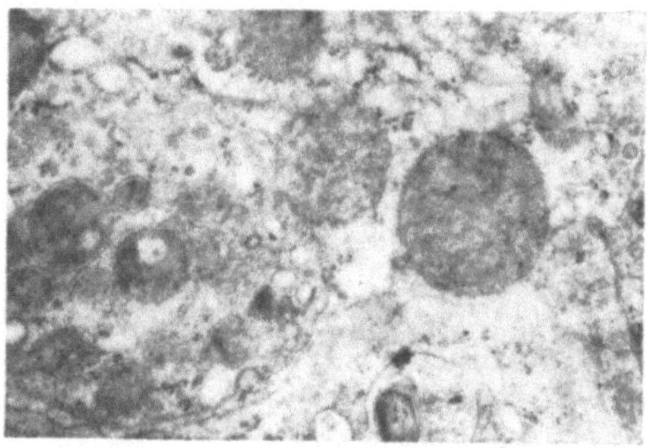

Abb. 1. Autophagolysosom im Zytoplasma einer Leberzelle. Vergrößerung 20000 × 2,3

Bei den Tieren der I. und II. Gruppen (140tägige freie Ernährung mit und ohne körperliche Belastung) unterscheidet sich das Bild wenig von den Kontrolltieren mit 20tägiger Versuchsdauer (Gruppe Ia). Veränderungen wurden aber bei den Tieren mit reduzierter Ernährung (Gruppe III) festgestellt. Hier gab es einerseits Überschuß an AFLS und andererseits an Zytolysomen (oder restliche Körperchen), in denen Strukturen fremder Organellen überhaupt nicht beobachtet werden konnten (Abb. 1). Bei Kombination der reduzierten Ernährung mit körperlicher Belastung (Gruppe II) wurden keine wesentlichen Unterschiede im ultrastrukturellen Bild festgestellt.

Von besonderem Interesse sind die Ergebnisse der biochemischen Untersuchungen (Abb. 2). Die reduzierte Ernährung (60% der freien Fütterung) wurde von einer erheblichen Aktivität der meisten Enzyme der Lysosomen in der Leber begleitet; insbesondere waren die Aktivitäten des Kathepsins und der sauren Ribonuclease erhöht (bis 180—200% vom Kontrollniveau). Etwas weniger (140—160%) erhöhte sich die Aktivität der sauren Desoxyribonuclease, β-Glucosidase, α-Galactosidase, β-Acetylglucosaminidase und der sauren Phosphatase. Die Aktivität der β-Galactosidase, β-Glucuronidase und der Arylsulfatase A und B erhöhte sich nur auf 115—125% des Kontrollniveaus.

Tabelle 1

Einfluß einer reduzierten Ernährung und körperlichen Belastung auf die nicht sedimentierte Aktivität der Leberlysosomen (nicht sedimentierte Aktivität in Prozent der Gesamtaktivität)

Gruppe	Enzyme						
	Saure Desoxyribonuclease	β-Glucosidase	β-Galactosidase	α-Galactosidase	Arylsulfatase A und B	Saure Phosphatase	N-acetylglucosaminidase
Freie Ernährung	26,6±1,4	15,0±1,8	28,0±2,0	13,3±2,1	2,6±0,2	18,6±0,8	1,5±0,2
Freie Ernährung und körperliche Belastung	27,2±1,4	13,5±0,7	27,0±1,9	12,0±0,4	2,0±0,1	17,6±0,7	1,4±0,2
P	0,05	0,05	0,05	0,05	0,05	0,05	0,05
Reduzierte Ernährung	28,4±1,3	15,5±4,1	32,2±1,6	19,4±1,4	4,7±0,3	13,2±2,5	3,9±0,4
P	0,05	0,05	0,05	0,05	0,001	0,05	0,001
Reduzierte Ernährung und körperliche Belastung	33,4±2,7	12,7±1,7	28,0±1,3	13,2±1,3	3,5±0,3	16,8±0,6	2,5±0,4
P	0,05	0,05	0,05	0,05	0,05	0,05	0,05

Es handelt sich um die Ergebnisse ($\bar{x} \pm s_{\bar{x}}$) von 8 Ratten pro Gruppe. P — im Vergleich mit der Kontrollgruppe.

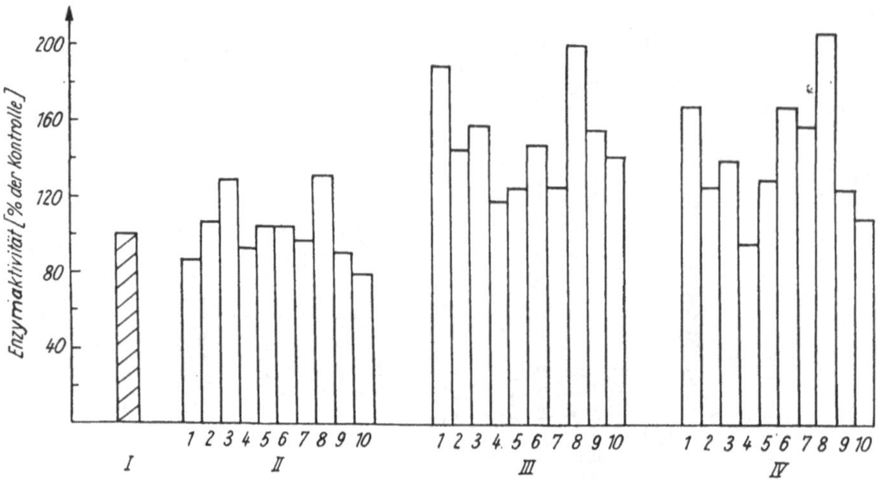

Abb. 2. Wirkung der reduzierten Ernährung und körperlichen Belastung auf die Aktivität der Leberlysosomen.
I — Freie Ernährung (Kontrolle); II — Freie Ernährung und körperliche Belastung; III — Reduzierte Ernährung; IV — Reduzierte Ernährung und körperliche Belastung
1. Saure Ribonuclease; 2. saure Desoxyribonuclease; 3. β-Glucosidase; 4. β-Glucuronidase; 5. α-Galactosidase; 6. β-Galactosidase; 7. Arylsulfatase A und B; 8. Kathepsin; 9. saure Phosphatase; 10. β-Acetylglucosaminidase

In der Aktivität der Enzyme der Leberlysosomen von Ratten waren wesentliche Veränderungen unter dem Einfluß der körperlichen Belastung bei freier Ernährung (Gruppe II) nicht festzustellen. Die Aktivitäten der untersuchten Enzyme der Leber der Tiere, die begrenztes Futter kombiniert mit körperlicher Belastung (Gruppe IV) erhielten, zeigten ebenso wie die von Tieren, die nur der reduzierten Ernährung unterworfen waren (Gruppe III) eine erhebliche Erhöhung (mit Ausnahme der β-Glucuronidase) aller Enzyme der Lysosomen, besonders des Kathepsins.

Bei der Untersuchung der Stabilität der Lysosomen-Membranen wurden keine wesentlichen Veränderungen in der nicht sedimentierbaren Aktivität der Marker-Enzyme (Tab. 1) festgestellt. Bei Ratten, die der reduzierten Ernährung mit oder ohne körperliche Belastung (Gruppen III und IV) unterzogen waren, war eine gewisse Erhöhung der nicht sedimentierbaren Aktivität einiger lysosomaler Enzyme zu verzeichnen.

Diskussion

Bei der ultrastrukturellen Untersuchung der Tiere der ersten Serie (20tägige Versuchsdauer, freie und eingeschränkte Ernährung) führt die körperliche Belastung zur Aktivierung des Lysosomensystems, die sich in der vermehrten Zahl der perinuklear verteilten Lysosomen ausdrückt.

Am 140. Tag sind die Veränderungen in den Gruppen mit reduzierter Ernährung ausgeprägter; die Aktivität der untersuchten lysosomalen Enzyme ist erhöht, und elektronenmikroskopisch ist nicht nur eine Erhöhung des AFLS, sondern auch der zytolysomen festzustellen.

Zieht man in Betracht, daß die freie Ernährung zum Auftreten von Fett-Tröpfchen in den Leberzellen führt, kann man annehmen, daß tatsächlich eine Überernährung vorliegt. Die erhaltenen Angaben über das Auftreten einer Autophagie zeigen, daß diese entweder physiologisch oder Zeichen eines beginnenden pathologischen Prozesses ist.

Es ist wichtig festzustellen, daß die morphologischen und die biochemischen Untersuchungen zu parallelen Ergebnissen führen. Die wesentlichsten Veränderungen in der Aktivität der lysosomalen Enzyme wurden bei den einer reduzierten Ernährung unterzogenen Tieren beobachtet; die körperliche Belastung beeinflußt die Aktivitätsveränderungen der untersuchten Enzyme nicht signifikant.

Summary

L. KRUSTEV, T. TASCHEV, A. POKROVSKIJ, W. TUTELJAN, I. APOSTOLOV, L. KRAWTSCHENKO, and A. POPOV: The effect of reduced diet and physical stress on liver lysosomes. Morphological and biochemical examinations

Groups of 15 rats each (I — non-reduced diet; II — non-reduced diet and physical stress; III — diet reduced by 40%; IV — reduced diet and physical stress) were examined after 20 and 140 days, respectively. The electron microscopic examination revealed that the most important changes had occurred in group III; there exists an excess of autophagolysosomes. The biochemical examinations show that the reduced diet (group III) also produces a considerable increase in activity of most of the lysosome enzymes in the liver.

The occurrence of autophagy evidences that this is either physiologically induced or the manifestation of a beginning pathological process.

Резюме

Л. Крыстев, Т. Ташев, А. Покровский, В. Тутелян, И. Апостолов, Г. Кравченко и А. Попов: Влияние редуцированного питания и физической нагрузки на лизосомы печени. Морфологические и биохимические исследования

Исследовались группы крыс из 15 животных в группе (I — свободное питание, II — свободное питание и физическая нагрузка, III — редуцированное на 40% питание, IV — редуцированное питание и физическая нагрузка) через 20 или 140 дней. При электронной микроскопии наибольшие изменения наблюдались в группе III; имеет место избыток автофаголизосом. Биохимические исследования показали, что редуцированное питание (группа III) сопровождается также значительным увеличением активности большинства лизосомальных энзимов печени.

Появление автофагии означает, что она является или Физиологическим или выражением начинающегося патологического процесса.

Literatur

[1] KRUSTEV, L. P., Archiv patologii, Moskau **35**, 52—57 (1973).

[2] KRUSTEV, L. P., T. A. TASHEV, A. A. POPOV, J. Z. APOSTOLOV, B. J. BOROV und M. S. STEFANOVA, Nahrung **20**, 597—603 (1976).

[3] LOWRY, O. H., u. a., J. biol. Chem. **193**, 265—275 (1951).

[4] POKROVSKIJ, A. A.: In Proc. 8. Internat. Congr. Nutrit., Prague 1969, S. 27—31, Herausgegeben von J. MAŠEK, K. OŠANCOVÁ u. D. R. CUTHBERTŠON; Excerpta Medica, Amsterdam 1970.

[5] POKROVSKIJ, A. A., u. V. A. TUTELJAN, Uspechi sovremennoi biologii **68**, 341—362 (1969).

[6] POKROVSKIJ, A. A. u. a., Dokl. Akad. Nauk, SSSR **205**, 1483—1487 (1972).

[7] POKROVSKIJ, A. A., u. L. P. KRUSTEV: Leber, Lysosomen und Ernährung (russisch). Herausgegeben von T. TASHEV, Isdat. BAN, Sofia 1977.

Dr. L. P. KRUSTEV, Institut für Ernährung, Sofia 31, Dimitar Nestorov 15, VR Bulgarien

Eingegangen 30. 8. 1977

Die Nahrung	22	3	1978	315–321

Hochschule für Lebensmittelindustrie Plovdiv, VR Bulgarien

Beständigkeit von S-Methylmethionin (Vitamin U) in Pufferlösungen und Pflanzensäften bei thermischer Behandlung

E. G. KOVATSCHEVA

Es wurde die Kinetik des thermischen Abbaus von S-Methylmethionins (MMS^+) in 0,02 M Citrat/Phosphat-Pufferlösungen bei pH 4,0, 6,0 und 8,0 sowie in Säften aus Sellerie, Tomaten Kohl und roter Rübe bei 50, 62, 74, 86, 98, 110 und 122 °C untersucht.
Durch die erhaltenen Versuchsdaten wurden die Reaktionsordnung des thermischen MMS^+-Abbaus zu Dimethylsulfid und Homoserin bestimmt und die Geschwindigkeitskonstanten, die Halbwertszeiten des Abbaus und die Aktivierungsenergien der in den erwähnten Pufferlösungen und Pflanzensäften verlaufenden Prozesse berechnet.

S-Methylmethionin (MMS^+; Vitamin U) ist ein biologisch aktiver Faktor mit nachgewiesener Antiulcuswirkung [1]. Das bedingt auch seine breite Verwendung in der medizinischen Praxis, und zwar nicht nur als synthetisches Salz [2], sondern auch in Form seines natürlichen Vorkommens in Pflanzen [2].

Bei der Untersuchung der Salze des S-Methylmethionins weisen TOENNIES u. a. [3] und später auch Mc RORIE u. a. [4] auf die hohe Thermolabilität der Verbindung hin. Nach LAVINE [5] wird die Art des thermischen Abbaus und die chemische Natur der Abbauprodukte hauptsächlich von der Zusammensetzung des Mediums bestimmt, in dem die Reaktion erfolgt. Der MMS^+-Abbau erfolgt in konzentrierten Säuren unter Bildung von Methionin und einem Methylderivat der entsprechenden Säure

$$(H_3C)_2S^+-CH_2-CH_2-\underset{\substack{|\\NH_2}}{CH}-COOH + HX \rightleftarrows H_3C-S-CH_2-CH_2-\underset{\substack{|\\NH_2}}{CH}-COOH + CH_3X + H^+ \quad (I)$$

und in wäßrigen Lösungen unter Bildung von Dimethylsulfid und Homoserin

$$(H_3C)_2S^+-CH_2-CH_2-\underset{\substack{|\\NH_2}}{CH}-COO^- \rightarrow (H_3C)_2S + HO-CH_2-CH_2-\underset{\substack{|\\NH_2}}{CH}-COOH \quad (II)$$

HIROAKA u. a. [6] sowie WILLIAMS u. a. [7] untersuchten den Einfluß der Temperatur und des pH-Wertes auf den Abbau von S-Methylmethionin in wäßrigen Lösungen und bewiesen, daß nicht nur die Temperatur, sondern auch der pH-Wert einen beträchtlichen Einfluß auf die Reaktionsgeschwindigkeit ausüben. Der Prozeß verläuft im alkalischen wesentlich intensiver als im sauren Medium.

Die thermische Unbeständigkeit der S-Methylsulfonsalze, die von der Bildung von Dimethylsulfid begleitet ist, wurde auch von anderen Autoren beobachtet, die das Aroma konservierter Produkte aus Tomaten, Kartoffeln und Mais untersuchten [8–11].

Die beobachtete hohe Thermolabilität des MMS^+ gab uns die Anregung zu einer gründlicheren Untersuchung seiner Beständigkeit unter verschiedenen Bedingungen

(Temperatur, Behandlungsdauer, pH-Wert und Zusammensetzung des Mediums) sowohl in Modellsystemen als auch in Pflanzensäften. Hauptziel der vorliegenden Arbeit ist die Untersuchung der kinetischen Parameter, die den thermischen Degradationsprozeß von MMS^+ charakterisieren. Sie sind für die Ermittlung der Bedingungen einer maximalen Erhaltung von MMS^+ bei der Konservierung der daran reichen pflanzlichen Quellen geeignet.

Experimenteller Teil

Untersuchung der thermischen Beständigkeit von MMS^+ in Pufferlösungen

Bei der Untersuchung der Beständigkeit von MMS^+ wurden MMSCl[1]-Lösungen in 0,02 M Citrat/Phosphat-Pufferlösungen mit pH-Werten von 4,0; 6,0 und 8,0 verwendet. Je 20 cm^3 der MMS^+-Lösungen mit einer Konzentration von 20 µg MMS^+/cm^3 wurden in Ampullen gefüllt (5 Parallelproben für jedes Regime), zugeschmolzen, temperiert und bei 50, 62, 74, 86, 98, 110 und 122 °C thermostatiert. Die Dauer des Erhitzens bei den einzelnen Proben richtete sich je nach dem Temperaturregime (siehe Abbildungen). Nach der thermischen Behandlung wurden die Ampullen für 10—15 min in Eis gelegt und anschließend in einem Rotationsverdampfer bei 50 °C zur Trockene eingedampft. Der Rückstand jeder Probe wurde in 1 cm^3 0,05 N Salzsäure aufgelöst, und je 25 µl der erhaltenen Lösungen wurden einer dünnschichtchromatographischen Trennung auf Silicagelplatten mit dem System n-Propanol/24% Ammoniak (6:4) unterworfen. Auf jedes Chromatogramm wurden parallel mit den thermisch behandelten Proben 25 µl Standardlösung mit einer Konzentration von 400 µg MMS^+/cm^3 aufgetragen. Nach dem Chromatographieren wurden die Platten getrocknet und in 1%iger Ninhydrin-Lösung (1,00 g Ninhydrin, 10 cm^3 Eisessig, Aceton auf 100 cm^3) entwickelt. 1 h nach dem Besprühen wurden die dem MMS^+ entsprechenden Flecke mit Methanol-Cadmiumreaktiv (0,20 g Cadmiumacetat, 2 cm^3 Wasser, Methanol auf 100 cm^3) eluiert und bei 506 nm mit einem Kolorimeter „Specol" (VEB Carl Zeiß, Jena, DDR) photometriert.

Untersuchung der thermischen Beständigkeit von MMS^+ in pflanzlichen Säften

Zur Untersuchung der thermischen MMS^+-Beständigkeit pflanzlicher Produkte wurden diese Verbindung enthaltende Pflanzensäfte verwendet. Je 20 cm^3 Saft aus Sellerie (Sorte „Pionier"; 45,5 µg MMS^+/cm^3; pH 4,05), Saft aus roten Tomaten (Sorte „Mekis"; 35,0 µg MMS^+/cm^3; pH 4,40), Saft aus roten Rüben (Sorte „Ägyptisch"; 21,4 µg MMS^+/cm^3; pH 6,20) und Saft aus Kohl (Sorte „Dabensko"; 30,1 µg MMS^+/cm^3; pH 6,15) wurden in Ampullen gegeben (je 5 Parallelproben für jedes Regime) und unter den schon erwähnten Bedingungen behandelt.

Die MMS^+-Menge in den ursprünglichen und thermisch behandelten Säfteproben wurde nach einem Verfahren bestimmt, das die Reinigung mit einem stark sauren Ionenaustauscher (Dowex 50 × 8) in Ammoniakform [12] und eine nachfolgende zweidimensionale Dünnschichtchromatographie auf Silikagel G mit den Laufmitteln Butanol/Aceton/24% Ammoniak (10:10:7) und n-Propanol/Ameisensäure/Wasser (20:1:5) beinhaltet.

Ergebnisse und Diskussion

Die erhaltenen Angaben über die thermischen Veränderungen der MMS^+-Konzentration in 0,02 M Citrat/Phosphat-Pufferlösungen erweisen sich als Reaktion 1. Ordnung. Dies ist aus dem linearen Verlauf des Logarithmus der Verhältnisse der MMS^+-Konzentrationen zu Beginn (MMS_0^+) und nach thermischer Behandlung (MMS_τ^+) bei den verschiedenen geprüften Temperaturen (50—122 °C) und pH-Werten (4,6 und 8) ersichtlich (Abb. 1—6). Zu derselben Schlußfolgerung gelangen WILILAMS u. a. [7],

[1] MMSCl wurde am Bach-Institut für Biochemie der Akademie der Wissenschaften der UdSSR, Moskau, synthesiert.

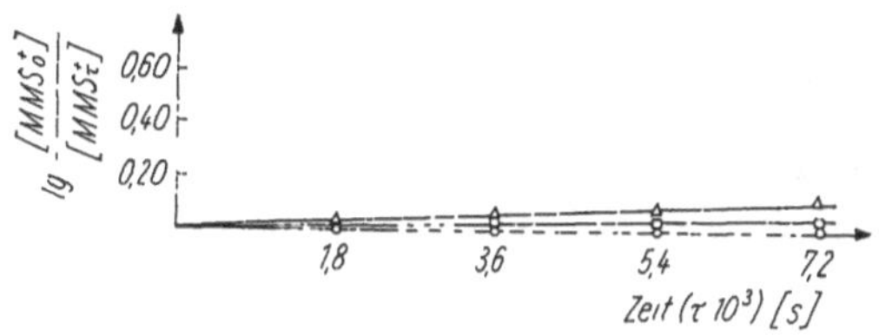

Abb. 1. Abhängigkeit von $\lg \frac{[MMS_0^+]}{[MMS_\tau^+]}$ beim thermischen MMS^+-Abbau (20 µg/cm³) in 0,02 M Citrat-Phosphat-Pufferlösungen bei 62 °C (○ = pH 4,0; □ = pH 6,0; △ = pH 8,0)

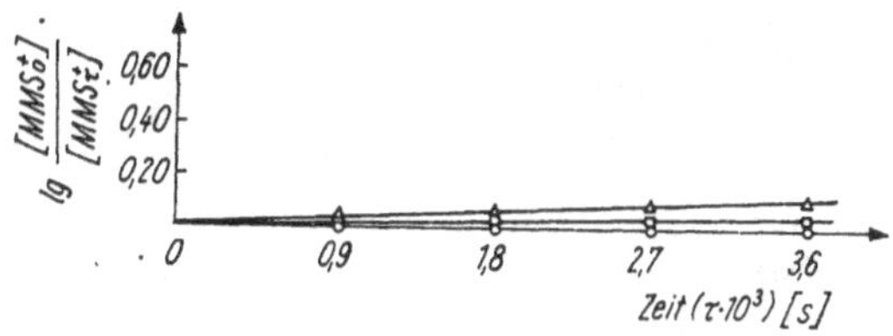

Abb. 2. MMS^+-Abbau bei 74 °C (vgl. Abb. 1)

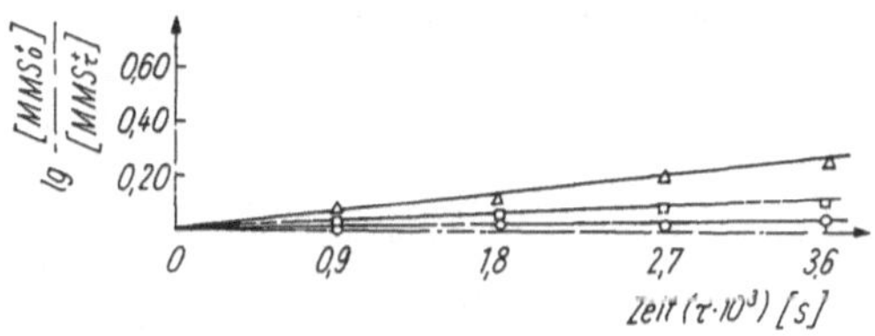

Abb. 3. MMS^+-Abbau bei 86 °C (vgl. Abb. 1)

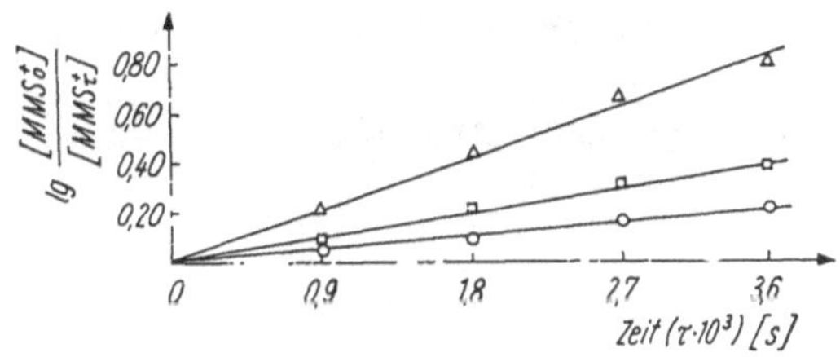

Abb. 4. MMS^+-Abbau bei 98 °C (vgl. Abb. 1)

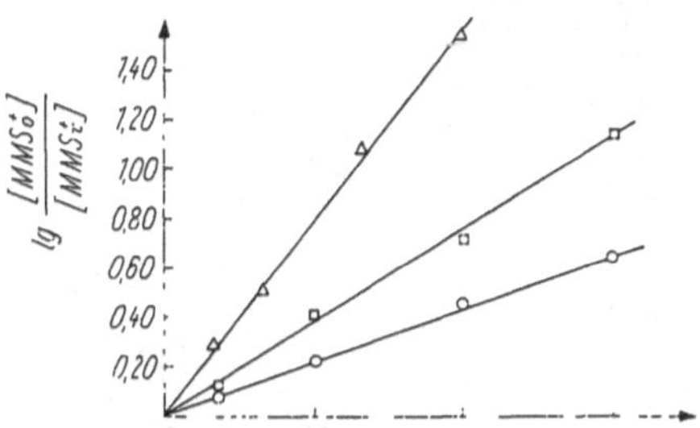

Abb. 5. MMS^+-Abbau bei 110 °C (vgl. Abb. 1)

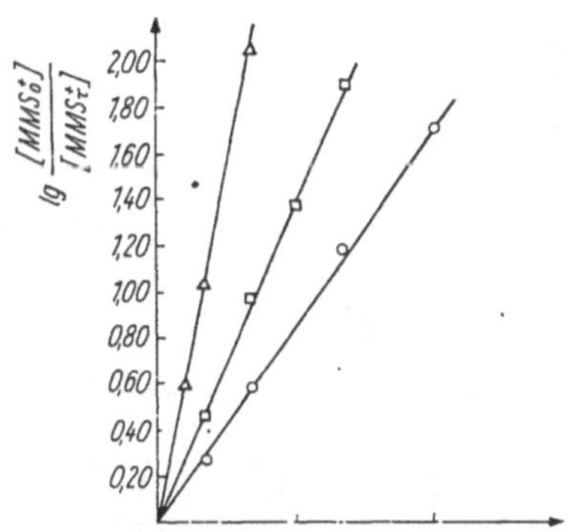

Abb. 6. MMS^+-Abbau bei 122 °C (vgl. Abb. 1)

indem sie die Kinetik der MMS^+-Degradation im Intervall von 82 bis 99 °C untersuchen. Ähnliche Schlüsse über die Ordnung der Reaktion kann man auch aus den geradlinigen kinetischen Abhängigkeiten ziehen, die bei der Untersuchung des MMS^+-Abbaus zu $(CH_3)_2S$ und Homoserin in Sellerie-, Tomaten-, Kohl- und Rote-Rüben-Säften erhalten wurden (Abb. 7—10). Deshalb wurden die den Prozeß charakterisierenden Parameter unter den Bedingungen einer Reaktion 1. Ordnung berechnet. Die Geschwindigkeitskonstanten (k) lassen sich aus dem Anstieg der Geraden bestimmen ($k = 2{,}3 \cdot \mathrm{tg}\alpha$; vgl. Abb. 1—10). Vergleicht man die beim thermischen MMS^+-Abbau in Pufferlösungen (Tab. 1) und in Pflanzensäften (Tab. 2) erhaltenen Werte, so sieht man, daß sie wesentlich von der Temperatur abhängen. Bei einer Erhöhung von 12 °C

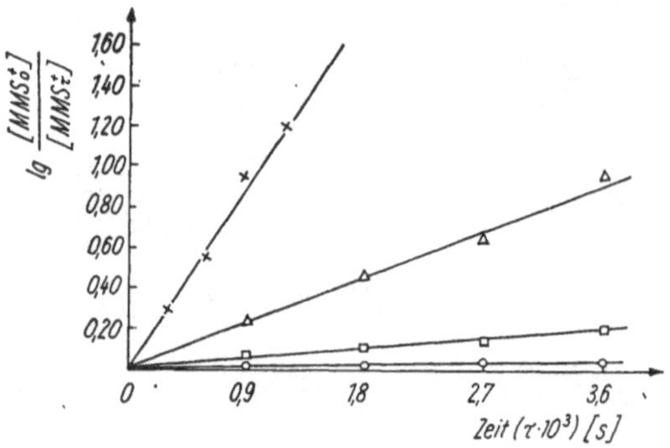

Abb. 7. Abhängigkeit von $\lg \frac{[MMS_0^+]}{[MMS_\tau^+]}$ von der Zeit beim thermischen MMS^+-Abbau in Selleriesaft (41,5 µg/cm³; pH 4,05) bei verschiedenen Temperaturen (○ = 86 °C; □ = 98 °C; △ = 110 °C; × = 122 °C)

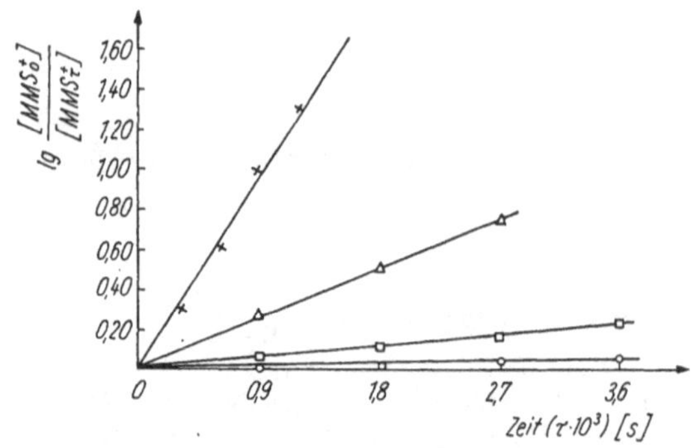

Abb. 8. MMS^+-Abbau in Tomatensaft (35,0 µg/cm³; pH 4,40) (vgl. Abb. 7)

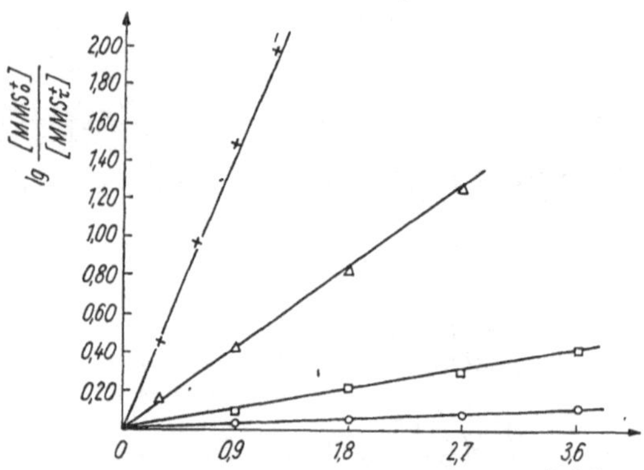

Abb. 9. MMS^+-Abbau in Kohlsaft (30,1 µg/cm³; pH 6,15) (vgl. Abb. 7)

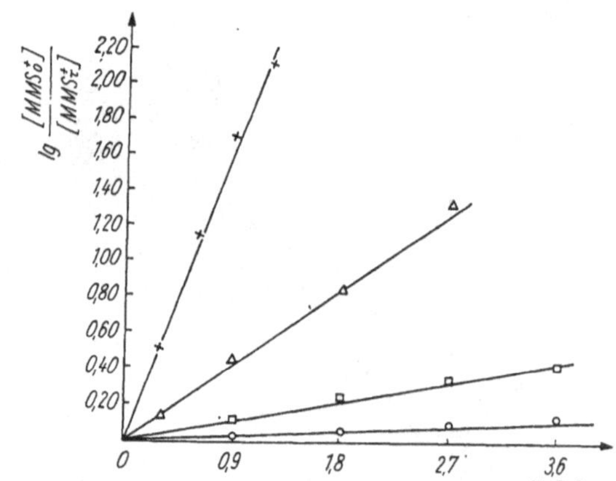

Abb. 10. MMS^+-Abbau in Rote-Rüben-Saft (21,4 µg/cm³; pH 6,20) (vgl. Abb. 7)

Tabelle 1

Geschwindigkeitskonstanten ($k \times 10^4$; in s^{-1}) des thermischen Abbaus von MMS^+ (20 µg/cm³) in 0,02 M Citrat-Phosphat-Pufferlösungen

pH	Temperatur [°C]						
	50	62	74	86	98	110	122
4,0	0	0	0	0,38	1,40	5,36	21,45
6,0	0	0,13	0,25	0,38	2,43	9,19	35,24
8,0	0	0,32	0,64	1,66	5,23	19,50	78,13

Tabelle 2
Geschwindigkeitskonstanten ($k \times 10^4$; in s^{-1})
des thermischen Abbaus von MMS^+ in einigen Pflanzensäften

Produkt	pH	Temperatur [°C]			
		86	98	110	122
1. Saft aus Sellerie, Sorte „Pionier", mit 41,5 µg MMS^+/cm^3	4,05	0,38	1,40	5,87	22,21
2. Saft aus Tomaten, Sorte „Mekis", mit 35,0 µg MMS^+/cm^3	4,40	0,38	1,53	6,38	24,51
3. Saft aus Kohl, Sorte „Dabcnsko", mit 30,1 µg MMS^+/cm^3	6,15	0,77	2,68	10,98	36,77
4. Saft aus roter Rübe, Sorte „Ägyptisch", mit 21,4 µg MMS/cm^3	6,20	0,89	2,80	10,98	42,13

im Bereich 50—122 °C erhöhen sich die Geschwindigkeitskonstanten auf jeweils den 1,9 bis 4,0fachen Wert bei Pufferlösungen und auf den 3,2 bis 4,2fachen Wert bei Pflanzensäften. Die Versuchsdaten zeigen, daß die Geschwindigkeitskonstante auch vom pH-Wert des Mediums abhängt. So steigt sie z.B. im Mittel bei einer pH-Zunahme von 4,0 auf 6,0 in Citrat-Phosphat-Pufferlösungen auf das 1,8fache und bei einer Änderung von 6,0 auf 8,0 um das 2,3fache. Beim MMS^+-Abbau in Pflanzensäften liegen die Zunahmen in gleicher Größenordnung. Bei einem Vergleich der Geschwindigkeitskonstanten der thermischen MMS^+-Degradation in Pufferlösungen und pflanzlichen Säften sind bei gleicher Temperatur, annähernd gleicher Konzentration und gleichem pH-Wert keine wesentlichen Unterschiede zu bemerken. Das berechtigt uns zu der Annahme, daß die Zusammensetzung des Mediums keinen wesentlichen Einfluß auf die Geschwindigkeit des Prozesses ausübt. Letztere Schlußfolgerung ist besonders wichtig, da die beim thermischen MMS^+-Abbau in Pufferlösungen erhaltenen Ergebnisse für eine Voraussage der Verluste bei der technologischen Bearbeitung der Pflanzensäfte mit genügender Zuverlässigkeit angewendet werden können.

Weiterhin wurden die Halbwertzeiten des Abbaues ($\tau_{1/2} = 0{,}693/k$ in s) und die Aktivierungsenergie (in kJ/mol) berechnet. Diese Größen können ebenfalls zur Charakterisierung der Reaktionsgeschwindigkeit verwendet werden. Die MMS^+-Halbwertszeiten nehmen bei thermischer Behandlung seiner Pufferlösungen (Tab. 3) und der Pflanzensäfte (Tab. 4) mit zunehmender Temperatur bei einem bestimmten pH-Wert ab. Die Abnahme ist bei niedrigen etwas schneller als bei hohen Temperaturen.

Tabelle 3
Halbwertzeiten ($\tau_{1/2} \times 10$; in s) der thermischen MMS^+-Degradation
in 0,02 M Citrat-Phosphat-Pufferlösungen

pH	Temperatur [°C]					
	62	74	86	98	110	122
4,0	∞	∞	18,24	4,95	1,29	0,32
6,0	53,31	27,72	9,00	2,85	0,75	0,20
8,0	21,66	10,83	4,18	1,33	0,35	0,09

Tabelle 4
Halbwertszeiten ($\tau_{1/2} \times 10$, in s) der thermischen MMS^+-Degradation in Pflanzensäften

Produkt	Temperatur [°C]			
	86	98	110	122
1. Selleriesaft (pH 4,05)	18,24	4,95	1,18	0,31
2. Tomatensaft (pH 4,40)	18,24	4,53	1,09	0,28
3. Kohlsaft (pH 6,15)	9,00	2,59	0,63	0,19
4. Rote-Rüben-Saft (pH 6,20)	7,79	2,48	0,63	0,16

Tabelle 5
Aktivierungsenergien der Reaktion des thermischen MMS^+-Abbaus in 0,02 M Citrat-Phosphat-Pufferlösungen

pH	MMS^+ [μg/cm³]	E [kJ/mol]
4,0	20,0	136,47
6,0	20,0	131,88
8,0	20,0	127,30

Tabelle 6
Aktivierungsenergien der Reaktion des thermischen MMS^+-Abbaus in einigen Pflanzensäften

Produkt	pH-Wert	MMS^+ [μg/cm³]	E [kJ/mol]
Selleriesaft	4,05	41,5	132,00
Tomatensaft	4,40	35,0	132,00
Kohlsaft	6,15	30,1	119,46
Rote-Rüben-Saft	6,20	21,4	127,48

Die Aktivierungsenergie des untersuchten Prozesses wurde nach der ARRHENIUS-Gleichung berechnet. Die erhaltenen Ergebnisse sind in den Tab. 5 und 6 dargestellt. Die für den thermischen Abbau von MMS^+ in Pflanzensäften aus Sellerie, Rüben, Kohl und Tomaten notwendigen Aktivierungsenergien stehen dem für denselben Prozeß in Citrat-Phosphat-Pufferlösungen berechneten Wert sehr nahe. Das beweist erneut die Annahme, daß die Zusammensetzung des Mediums keinen wesentlichen Einfluß auf die Reaktionsgeschwindigkeit ausübt.

Die durchgeführten Untersuchungen über die Beständigkeit des MMS^+ zeigen, daß die Geschwindigkeit des thermischen Abbaus von der Temperatur, der Einwirkungszeit und vom pH-Wert des Mediums bestimmt wird.

Summary

E. G. KOVATSCHEVA: Stability of S-Methylmethionine in Buffer Solutions and Vegetable Juices in the Course of Thermal Treatment

The kinetic and thermal decomposition of S-methylmethionine (MMS^+) in 0,02 M citrate-phosphate buffer solutions with pH 4,00, 6,00, 8,00 and vegetable juices of celery, tomatoes, cabbage and beetroot at temperatures of 50, 62, 74, 86, 98, 110 and 122 °C was studied.

The reaction order of thermal degradation of MMS^+ to dimethylsulfide and homoserine was established. The rate constants, half time periods and activation energies of the reactions in buffer solutions and vegetable juices were calulated.

Резюме

Е. Г. Ковачева: Устойчивость S — метилметионина в буферных растворах и растительных соках при термической обработке

Изучена кинетика термического распада S — метилметионона (MMS^+) в 0,02 m цитратно-фосфатных растворах с pH 4,00, 6,00, и 8,00 и в растителных соках из сельдерея, томатов, капусты и салатной свеклы при температуре 50, 62, 74, 86, 98, 110 и 122 °C.

В результате опытных данных определен порядок реакции термической деградации MMS^+ до диметилсульфида и гомосерина, вычислены скоростные константы, период полураспада и активирующая энергия процесса, протекающего в указанных и буферных растительных соках.

Literatur

[1] Bukin, V. N., und G. N. Hutschua, Uspechi biol. chimii **10**, 184 (1969).

[2] Bukin, V. N., und V. E. Anisimova (Herausgeber), Vitamin U (S-Methylmethionin). Priroda, svojstva, primenenie. Nauka, Moskva 1973.

[3] Toennies, G., und J. J. Kolb, J. Amer. chem. Soc. **67**, 849 (1945).

[4] McRorie, R. A., G. L. Sutherland, M. S. Lewis, A. D. Barton, M. R. Glasener und W. Shive, J. Amer. chem. Soc. **76**, 115 (1954).

[5] Lavine, T. F., und N. F. Floyd, J. biol. Chem. **207**, 97 (1954).

[6] Hiroaka, E., und T. Kishi, Vitamins **28**, 389 (1963).

[7] Williams, M. P., und P. E. Nelson, J. Food Sci. **39**, 457 (1974).

[8] Miers, J. C., J. agric. Food. Chem. **14**, 419 (1966).

[9] Quadagni, D. G., J. C. Miers und D. Venstrom, Food Technology **22**, 71 (1968).

[10] Gumbmann, M. R., und H. K. Burr, J. agric. Food Chem. **12**, 404 (1964).

[11] Bills, D. D., und T. W. Keenan, J. agric. Food Chem. **16**, 643 (1968).

[12] Kovatscheva, E., und Y. G. Popova, Nahrung **21**, 465 (1977).

Elena G. Kovatscheva, Hochschule für Lebensmittelindustrie, Plovdiv, Boul. Lenin 26, VR Bulgarien

Eingegangen 2. 9. 1977

Die Nahrung	22	3	1978	323–329

Hochschule für Lebensmittelindustrie Plovdiv, VR Bulgarien

Beständigkeit von S-Methylmethionin bei Konservierung seiner Pflanzenquellen durch Sterilisation

E. G. KOVATSCHEVA

Untersucht wurde die Beständigkeit des Antiulcusfaktors S-Methylmethionin (MMS^+) während der Sterilisation seiner Pflanzenquellen (Sellerie, rote Rüben, Himbeeren, Tomaten und Mais) nach den in Bulgarien üblichen technologischen Regimen und unter Bedingungen, die auf die hohe Thermolabilität des MMS^+ eingestellt waren.
Es werden Bedingungen empfohlen, die die maximale Erhaltung von MMS^+ bei der Herstellung von konservierten Produkten aus den genannten Obst- und Gemüsearten gewährleisten.

Die Ergebnisse der bisher durchgeführten Untersuchungen über die thermische Degradation des Antiulcusfaktors S-Methylmethionin (MMS^+) zeigen seine hohe Thermolabilität. Die Geschwindigkeit seines Abbaus wird von der Temperatur, der Behandlungsdauer und dem pH-Wert des Mediums bestimmt, ohne daß sie von der Zusammensetzung des Lösungsmittels wesentlich beeinflußt wird [1–3].

Diese Daten berechtigen uns zu der Annahme, daß die biologische Vollwertigkeit der konservierten Naturprodukte in bezug auf MMS^+ hauptsächlich von den Bedingungen der technologischen Behandlung bestimmt wird. Untersuchungen zur Beständigkeit von MMS^+ während der Sterilisation seiner Pflanzenquellen und die Ermittlung der geeignetsten Bedingungen zu seiner maximalen Erhaltung beim Konservieren sind deshalb von besonderem Interesse.

Experimenteller Teil

Die Herstellung von sterilisierten Produkten aus Pflanzenquellen mit hohem MMS^+-Gehalt wie Sellerie, Rote Rüben, Tomaten, Himbeeren und Mais erfolgte entsprechend den in Bulgarien üblichen technologischen Regimen [4], sowie unter Bedingungen, die die hohe Thermolabilität des MMS^+ berücksichtigen.

Saft aus Sellerie. Das Rohgut (Sorte „Pionier") wurde gemäß der gebräuchlichen Technologie zu 5 mm großen Teilchen gemahlen, und es wurden 25% Wasser, 1 g/kg L-Ascorbinsäure und 4 g/kg Citronensäure zugesetzt. Ein Teil von dem so zubereiteten Gemisch (15,20 kg) wurde 10–12 min mit indirektem Dampf bei 97–98 °C behandelt. Die Masse wurde durch Umrühren bis 50 °C innerhalb von 45 min abgekühlt, und daraus erhielt man durch Pressen 8,70 kg Saft und 5,80 kg pflanzliches Preßgut.

Damit die thermische Degradation des MMS^+ beim Entziehen des Selleriesaftes vermieden wird, wurde die Sellerie einem enzymatischen Abbau unterworfen. Eine bestimmte Menge der Pflanzenmischung (15,20 kg) wurde 1 h bei 42–44 °C mit 1 g/kg mazerierendem Präparat „Rohament" (Röhm und Haas, BRD) behandelt. Danach wurde die Masse gepreßt, und es wurden 9,70 kg Saft und 5,40 kg Preßgut erhalten.

Der nach beiden Arten entzogene Saft mit pH 4,0 wurde bei 98 °C in Flaschen von 250 cm^3 10, 15, 20 bzw. 30 min sterilisiert. Die Temperaturveränderung in den Flaschen wurde mit Kupfer-Konstantan-Thermoelementen verfolgt.

Saft aus roter Rübe. Der Saft wurde nach zwei Verfahren entzogen: a) Durch Pressen der 30 min gekochten Rübenportionen von 20 kg der Sorte „Ägyptisch" mit Zusatz von 20% Wasser; die Saftausbeute betrug 57–60%. b) Durch Mahlen des Rohgutes zu 5 mm großen Teilchen und durch Pressen der erhaltenen Masse (Saftausbeute 76–78%).

Der pH-Wert des Rübensaftes wurde durch Zusatz von Citronensäure auf 4,0 gebracht, und der Saft wurde bei 98 °C 10, 15, 20 und 30 min sterilisiert.

Saft aus Himbeeren wurde durch Zerkleinern und Pressen des Rohgutes gewonnen. Nach seiner enzymatischen Klärung wurde der Saft mit pH 3,8 in Flaschen von 250 cm^3 10 min bei 98 °C sterilisiert.

Konservierte Produkte aus Tomate. Die sterilisierten Produkte aus grünen und roten Tomaten (Sorten „Chicco", „Ventura" und „Mekis") wurden nach den bei uns üblichen technologischen Instruktionen zubereitet. Beim Konservieren der grünen Tomaten wurde das Gut in Gläser (Typ „Omnia") gegeben und mit essigsaurem Aufguß versehen. Den roten Tomaten setzten wir einen aus dem entsprechenden Rohgut gewonnenen Saft zu. Die Sterilisation der grünen Tomaten mit pH 4,0–4,1 erfolgte bei 98 °C-10 min und die der roten Tomaten (pH 4,4–4,6) 30 min.

Aus roten Tomaten (Sorte „Mekis") gewannen wir Saft durch Mahlen, Blanchieren (5 min, 86 °C) und Passieren des Rohgutes. Das erhaltene Produkt wurde in Flaschen (250 cm^3) gegeben und 30 min bei 98 °C behandelt.

Konservierte Maisprodukte. Die Körner von süßem Mais (Sorte „Jubileumsmais") wurden in Dosen (250 cm^3) gegeben. Einen Teil der Proben begossen wir mit salzigem, einen anderen Teil mit süßem Aufguß. Die Sterilisation dauerte 20 min bei 120 °C.

Die Aufbewahrung von Sellerie-, Tomaten- und Rote-Rüben-Säften erfolgte unter den üblichen Lagerbedingungen und betrug 12 Monate.

Der MMS^+-Gehalt wurde in allen Pflanzenproben nach einem Verfahren ermittelt, das eine ionenaustauschchromatographische Reinigung von MMS^+ auf Dowex (NH_4^+-Form) [5] und nachfolgende zweidimensionale Dünnschichtchromatographie auf Silikagel G mit den Systemen 1 (n-Butanol: Aceton: 4%-Ammoniak = 10:10:7) und 2 (n-Propanol: Ameisensäure: Wasser = 20:1:5) beinhaltet.

Ergebnisse und Diskussion

Beim Studium der Verluste an MMS^+ während der Gewinnung von sterilisierten Produkten aus Sellerie nach der in der Produktion üblichen Technologie wurde festgestellt, daß bei der Anfangsbehandlung des Rohgutes innerhalb von 10–12 min bei 98 °C der MMS^+-Gehalt um 41,3% abnimmt (Tab. 1). Diese hohen Verluste sind nicht nur auf die Hochtemperaturbehandlung der Sellerie während 10 min., sondern hauptsächlich auf deren langsames Abkühlen zurückzuführen, bei dem die Temperatur der Masse noch 25–30 min lang über 80 °C bleibt. Beim enzymatischen Abbau des Gutes

Tabelle 1
Veränderungen des MMS^+-Gehalts bei der Behandlung von Sellerie

Art des Produktes und der Behandlung	Trockensubstanz [%]	MMS^+-Gehalt	
		[mg je 100 g Rohprodukt]	[mg je 100 g Trockensubstanz]
1. Sellerie; Sorte „Pionier"	10,7	7,5	70,0
2. Thermisch behandelte Sellerie (10–12 min bei 98 °C)	9,5	3,9	41,1
3. Enzymatisch behandelte Sellerie (60 min bei 42 °C)	7,9	5,1	64,6

innerhalb 1 h bei 42—44 °C mit 1 g/kg mazerierendem Präparat „Rohament" betragen die Verluste nur 7,8% (Tab. 1), womit auch die Gewinnung eines an MMS^+ um 50% reicheren Saftes im Vergleich zum Rohgut nach thermischer Behandlung zu erklären ist (Tab. 2). Deshalb ist es notwendig, einen enzymatischen Abbau des Rohgutes beim Gewinnen von Selleriesaft herbeizuführen. Wenn dagegen eine thermische Behandlung erfolgt, ist das erhaltene pflanzliche Gemisch schnell während 5 min auf 60—65 °C abzukühlen.

Tabelle 2
Veränderungen des MMS^+-Gehalts bei der Konservierung von Selleriesaft

Art der Gewinnung	Trocken-substanz [%]	MMS^+-Gehalt [mg je 100 g Rohprodukt]	MMS^+-Gehalt [mg je 100 g Trockensubstanz]
Saft aus thermisch behandeltem Rohgut			
1. Vor der Sterilisation	5,3	4,2	79,2
2. Sterilisiert bei 98 °C			
a) 10 min	5,2	3,5	67,4
b) 15 min	5,2	3,2	61,5
c) 20 min	5,3	2,9	54,7
d) 30 min	5,4	2,4	14,4
Saft aus enzymatisch behandeltem Rohgut			
1. Vor der Sterilisation	5,0	5,7	114,0
2. Sterilisiert bei 98 °C			
a) 10 min	5,0	4,9	98,0
b) 15 min	5,2	4,5	86,5
c) 20 min	5,2	4,0	76,9
d) 30 min	5,4	3,3	61,1

Die Sterilisation des nach beiden Verfahren erhaltenen Saftes (pH 4,0) erfolgte bei 98 °C während 10, 15, 20 bzw. 30 min, um den Einfluß der Behandlungsdauer auf die MMS^+-Verluste zu ermitteln. Die erhaltenen Ergebnisse zeigen, daß die Verluste bei enzymatisch behandeltem Rohgut durch die Sterilisation von 14,4% (10 min) auf 23,1% (15 min), 31,8% (20 min) bzw. 45,2% (30 min) ansteigen (Tab. 2). Zum Vergleichen der Effektivität der verschiedenen Zeiten wurden die Sterilisationseffekte nach Kyslink [6] für Produkte mit pH-Werten im sauren Bereich und einem Gefälle der Abtötungszeitkurve $Z = 15$ °C berechnet. Nach dem erwähnten Autor wird die Sterilität der Produkte bei einem Effekt erreicht, der wenigstens 2,5mal größer ist als der theoretisch als 1 angenommene. Aus den Werten der Sterilisationseffekte (Tab. 3) bei einer 10 min—2,40 min und 15 min—5,71 min dauernden Behandlung ist zu ersehen, daß die thermische Behandlung während 15 min bei 98 °C die beste Sterilität des Selleriesaftes gewährleistet. Das wird auch durch die Daten der mikrobiologischen Analyse bestätigt. Die eingeführten Sterilisationsbedingungen, auf die hohe Thermolabilität des MMS^+ eingestellt, müssen peinlichst eingehalten werden, da eine unwesentliche Verlängerung des Prozesses zu beträchtlichen Verlusten an MMS^+ im Produkt führen kann, ohne daß dessen Qualität daran gewinnt.

Tabelle 3
Sterilisationseffekt nach KYSLINK [6] für Produkte mit pH-Werten im sauren Bereich und einem Gefälle der Abtötungszeitkurve Z = 15 °C

Sterilisationsdauer [min]	Sterilisationseffekt [min]	
	für Selleriesaft mit pH 4,0	für Saft aus roten Rüben mit pH 4,0
10	2,40	2,31
15	5,71	5,50
20	13,75	12,90
30	29,29	29,90

Auf Grund der Versuchsdaten empfehlen wir zur Gewinnung von Saft aus roten Rüben mit einem hohen MMS+-Gehalt die Entziehung des Saftes durch Pressen der bis auf 4—5 mm Größe gemahlenen Teilchen des Rohgutes (Saftausbeute 76—78%). In diesem Falle liegen keine MMS+-Verluste als Folge der thermischen Degradation vor, und der entzogene Saft (pH 6,0) ist 2,5mal reicher an MMS+ als das Produkt, das durch Pressen der 30 min auf 98 °C erhitzten Rüben erhalten wird (Tab. 4). Die Saftausbeute ist dabei um 15—20% größer. Im Laufe der Sterilisation des angesäuerten Rübensaftes in Flaschen (pH 4,0) sind die festgestellten Verluste an MMS+ in derselben Größenord-

Tabelle 4
Veränderungen des MMS+-Gehalts bei konservierten Produkten aus roten Rüben, Himbeeren und Mais

Art des Produktes und Behandlungsverfahren	Trockensubstanz [%]	MMS+-Gehalt	
		[mg je 100 g Rohprodukt]	[mg je 100 g Trockensubstanz]
Rote Rübe			
1. Rohgut Sorte „Ägyptisch")	14,0	4,0	28,6
2. Saft, entzogen durch Pressen der gemahlenen Rübe	7,8	4,4	56,4
a) derselbe Saft, pH 4,0, 10 min bei 98 °C sterilisiert	7,8	3,8	48,7
b) derselbe Saft, pH 4,0, 15 min bei 98 °C sterilisiert	8,0	3,5	43,8
c) derselbe Saft, pH 4,0, 30 min bei 98 °C sterilisiert	8,0	2,6	32,5
3. Thermisch behandelte Rübe 30 min, 98 °C	13,1	2,9	22,2
4. Saft, der thermisch behandelten Rübe entzogen	8,3	1,8	22,0
Himbeeren			
1. Rohgut	11,3	3,2	28,3
2. Nichtsterilisierter Saft	10,0	3,4	34,0
3. 10 min bei 98 °C sterilisierter Saft	10,0	3,0	30,0
Mais			
1. Rohgut (Sorte „Jubiläumsmais")	22,1	8,0	36,2
2. Nichtsterilisierte Konserve	16,2	5,3	32,7
3. 20 min bei 120 °C sterilisierte Konserve	16,0	0	0

nung wie beim Selleriesaft. Bei einer Sterilisationsdauer von 10 min betragen sie 13,6%, bei 15 min 22,2%, und bei 30 min 42,4% (Tab. 4). Es ist ersichtlich, daß die Art des Gutes keinen wesentlichen Einfluß auf den Grad der Verluste an MMS^+ ausübt. Wenn annähernd gleiche Werte der Sterilisationseffekte der angewandten Bedingungen (Tab. 3) in Betracht gezogen werden, so ergeben sich für die Konservierung des Rübensaftes die gleichen Bedingungen wie bei der Sterilisation des Selleriesaftes (15 min bei 98 °C).

Die Ergebnisse über den Gehalt an MMS^+ in den Tomatenkonserven zeigen, daß die aus grünen Tomaten gewonnenen Produkte reicher an MMS^+ sind als die aus roten (Tab. 5). Das ist hauptsächlich darauf zurückzuführen, daß bei der Herstellung von

Tabelle 5
Veränderungen des MMS^+-Gehalts bei konservierten Produkten aus Tomaten

Rohgut und Art des konservierten Produktes	Vor der Sterilisation			Nach der Sterilisation (10 min, 98 °C)		
	Trocken-substanz [%]	[mg MMS^+ je 100 g konserv. Produkt]	[mg MMS^+ je 100 g Trocken-substanz]	Trocken-substanz [%]	[mg MMS^+ je 100 g konserv. Produkt]	[mg MMS^+ je 100 g Trocken-Substanz]
Eingesäuerte grüne Tomaten						
a) Sorte „Chicco"	8,0	3,4	42,5	8,0	2,8	35,0
b) Sorte „Ventura"	7,0	2,4	34,3	7,0	2,0	28,6
c) Sorte „Mekis"	7,0	3,3	47,1	7,2	2,9	40,3
Ganze rote Tomaten						
a) Sorte „Chicco"	8,0	4,0	50,0	8,2	2,0	24,4
b) Sorte „Ventura"	6,8	2,8	41,2	7,0	1,5	21,4
c) Sorte „Mekis"	7,0	4,0	57,1	7,3	2,1	28,8
Saft aus roten Tomaten Sorte „Mekis"	7,2	4,0	55,5	7,4	2,1	28,4

Alle Daten in den Tabellen sind das Ergebnis von drei parallel durchgeführten Versuchen

eingesäuerten grünen Tomaten die Sterilisation gemäß den technologischen Forderungen bei 98 °C 10 min dauert, während sie sich bei Konserven aus roten Tomaten (pH 4,4—4,6) auf 30 min erstreckt. Diese 3mal längere Dauer des Prozesses bedingt auch den niedrigeren MMS^+-Gehalt in den Fertigprodukten aus roten Tomaten. Aus den Versuchsdaten ist auch zu ersehen, daß die Verluste während der Sterilisation der Tomaten bei 10 min Erhitzungsdauer durchschnittlich 14,3% gegenüber 49,5% bei 30 min betragen. Dabei werden diese Werte kaum von den verschiedenen Sorten des Produktes beeinflußt.

Bei der Gewinnung von Saft aus roten Tomaten wurden während des Blanchierens des Rohgutes bei 86 °C während 5 min 5—6% Verluste an MMS^+ festgestellt. Bei der darauffolgenden Sterilisation bei 98 °C während 30 min nehmen sie wesentlich zu und erreichen 49,2% der MMS^+-Menge im frischen Saft.

Bei der Herstellung von Himbeersaft beträgt die Abnahme des MMS^+ nur 11,8% im Vergleich zum Rohgut. Diese geringen Verluste sind auf die kurzdauernde Sterilisation des Produktes — 10 min bei 98 °C — zurückzuführen, die durch den hohen Säuregehalt des Himbeersaftes (pH 3,8) bestimmt wird. In Konserven aus süßem

Mais (pH 6), 20 min auf 120 °C erhitzt) wird kein MMS^+ mehr festgestellt (Tab. 4), obwohl das Rohgut 2—3mal reicher an MMS^+ ist als das von Himbeeren.

Aus den oben behandelten Fällen ist ersichtlich, daß der Grad der MMS^+-Verluste bei sterilisierten Produkten aus verschiedenen Früchten und Gemüsearten ausschließlich von den Bedingungen der Hochtemperatursterilisation bestimmt wird und nicht wesentlich von der Natur des Rohgutes abhängig ist.

Während der Aufbewahrung der sterilisierten Produkte — Säfte aus Sellerie, roten Rüben und Tomaten 12 Monate unter den üblichen Lagerbedingungen (Abb. 1) — ist eine Zunahme der MMS^+-Verluste zu beobachten, die 4—5% je 2 Monate beträgt. Am Ende der einjährigen Periode ist der Gehalt an MMS^+ um 20 bis 26% in den drei untersuchten Produkten vermindert.

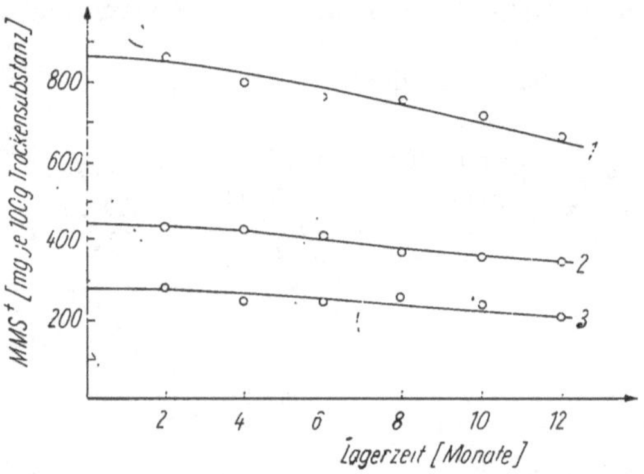

Abb. 1. Veränderung des MMS^+-Gehalts beim Aufbewahren von sterilisierten Säften während 12 Monaten. 1. Selleriesaft; 2. Saft aus roten Rüben; 3. Saft aus Tomaten

Schlußfolgerungen

Zur Gewinnung von Produkten mit einem hohem MMS^+-Gehalt aus üblichen Obst- und Gemüsequellen im sterilisierten Zustand sind folgende Bedingungen am zweckmäßigsten:

1. Der Saft aus Sellerie ist durch enzymatischen Abbau des Rohgutes mit einem mazerierenden Enzympräparat innerhalb 1 h bei 42—44 °C anstatt einer Entziehung nach thermischer Behandlung während 10—12 min bei 98 °C zu gewinnen. Die Konservierung des Selleriesaftes mit pH 4,0 soll 15 min bei 98 °C erfolgen.

2. Ein an MMS^+ wesentlich reicherer Saft (2,5mal) aus roten Rüben läßt sich durch Pressen des gemahlenen Gutes erzeugen. Das Erhitzen der Rübe während 30 min bei 89 °C ist zu vermeiden. Die Sterilisation des Saftes mit pH 4,0 soll bei 98 °C nicht länger als 15 min dauern.

3. Als Quellen des MMS^+ können auch andere sterilisierte Produkte aus an MMS^+ reichen Produkten wie Tomaten, Himbeeren und Erdbeeren verwendet werden.

4. Die Verluste an MMS^+ bei thermischer Behandlung seiner Pflanzenquellen werden hauptsächlich von den Bedingungen der Erhitzung bestimmt, ohne daß die Zusammensetzung dabei wesentlich mitbestimmend ist. Bei einer Behandlungsdauer von 10 min bei 98 °C betragen die Verluste 11,6—16,1%, von 20 min 31,0—32,5% und von 30 min 40,6—51,2% für die untersuchten Obst- und Gemüsearten.

5. Die sterilisierten Produkte — Säfte aus Sellerie, roten Rüben und Tomaten — weisen eine gute Stabilität des MMS^+ bei ihrer Aufbewahrung während eines Jahres in Räumen ohne Temperaturregulierung auf. Die Verluste überschreiten hierbei nicht 26%.

Summary

E. G. Kovatscheva: Stability of S-methylmethionine during conservation by sterilization of its vegetable origins

The stability of the antiulcer factor S-methylmethionine (MMS^+) was studied in the course of sterilization of its vegetable origins as celery, beetroot, raspberry, tomatoes, and maize according to the technological treatment generally used in Bulgaria, and on conditions, adapted to its high thermolability. As a result of this investigation conditions were recommended providing for a maximum preser vation of MMS^+ during conservation of the above-mentioned vegetables and fruits.

Резюме

Е. Г. Ковачева: Устойчивость S — Метилметионина при консервировании его растительных источников с помощью стерилизации

Изучена устойчивость противоязвенного фактора S — метилметионина (MMS^+) в процессе стрерилизации его растительных источников (сельдерея, салатной свелы, томатов и кукурузы) при технологических режимах, обычно применяемых в Болгарии и при условиях, соответствующих его высокой термолабильности. Предложены условия, обеспечивающие максимальное сохранение MMS^+ при получении консервированных продуктов вышеупомянутых плодов и овощей.

Literatur

[1] Hiroaka, E., u. T. Kishi, Vitamins **28**, 347 (1963).
[2] Williams, M., P., u. P. E. Nelson, J. Food Sci. **39**, 457 (1974).
[3] Kovatscheva, E. G., Nahrung, **22**, 315 (1978).
[4] Sbornik technologic instrukcii za proizvodstvo na plodovi i zelentschukovi konservi. t. 2. DSO „Bulgarplod", Sofia (1971).
[5] Kovatscheva, E. G., u. Y. G. Popova, Nahrung **21**, 465 (1977).
[6] Kyslink, V., Sbornik Vysoke Skoly Chemikotechnologicke v Praze. Praze (1957).

Elena G. Kovatscheva, Hochschule für Lebensmittelindustrie Plovdiv, Boul. „Lenin" 26, VR Bulgarien

Eingegangen 2. 9. 1977

Die Nahrung	22	3	1978	331–334

Hochschule für Lebensmittelindustrie Plovdiv, VR Bulgarien

Beständigkeit von S-Methylmethionin in Pufferlösungen und pflanzlichen Produkten bei ihrer Gefrierkonservierung

E. G. Kovatšcheva

Untersucht wurde die Beständigkeit von S-Methylmethionin (MMS^+) in Citrat-Phosphat-Pufferlösungen mit pH 4,0, 6,0 und 8,0 und in Pflanzensäften aus Sellerie und roten Rüben (in Ampullen) innerhalb von 12 Monaten bei +2, −13 und −18 °C. Außerdem wurde seine Beständigkeit bein Gefrieren und Aufbewahren seiner gefrorenen Pflanzenquellen (Sellerie, Blumenkohl, Himbeeren u. a.) bei −18 °C verfolgt.

Die erhaltenen Ergebnisse berechtigen uns, die Gefrierkonservierung als das geeignetste Konservierungsverfahren für die maximale Erhaltung von MMS^+ in seinen Pflanzenquellen zu empfehlen.

Die Thermolabilität des S-Methylmethionins (MMS^+), die den hohen Prozentsatz der Verluste dieses aktiven Faktors bei der Konservierung seiner Naturquellen durch Sterilisation [1] bestimmt, gab uns Anlaß zur Untersuchung seiner Beständigkeit bei niedrigen Temperaturen. Ziel der Untersuchung ist es, die geeignetsten Bedingungen für eine bessere Erhaltung des MMS^+ bei der Konservierung seiner reichen pflanzlichen Quellen zu finden, die nicht nur im frischen, sondern oft auch im bearbeiteten Zustand verbraucht werden.

Experimenteller Teil

Beständigkeit des MMS^+ in Pufferlösungen und Pflanzensäften bei niedrigen Temperaturen

Citrat-Phosphat-Pufferlösungen (0,02 M) von MMS-Cl mit einer Konzentration von 20 µg MMS^+/cm^3 und pH 4,0, 6,0 und 8,0 wurden in 20 cm^3-Ampullen gegeben und während 12 Monaten bei +2, −13 und −18 °C aufbewahrt. Unter gleichen Bedingungen wurden auch Säfte aus Sellerie (pH 4,0) und roten Rüben (pH 6,1) aufbewahrt, die 2 min bei 98 °C thermisch vorbehandelt wurden. Jeden zweiten Monat wurde die Zusammensetzung von Proben aus den MMS^+ enthaltenden Pufferlösungen und Pflanzensäften analysiert und mit der Zusammensetzung frisch erhaltener MMS^+-Standardlösungen verglichen. Die Menge des MMS^+ wurde nach Methoden bestimmt, die in einer früheren Mitteilung [2] beschrieben wurden.

Beständigkeit des MMS^+ bei der Gefrieraufbewahrung seiner Pflanzenquellen

Das Gefrieren und Aufbewahren der an MMS^+ reichen Naturprodukte erfolgte unter Produktionsbedingungen nach den in Bulgarien üblichen technologischen Regimen [3].

Selleriesaft, erhalten nach dem thermischen Abbau des Rohgutes [1], wurde in Plastikbeuteln von 250 cm^3 innerhalb 2,5–3,0 h in Gefrierräumen bei −18 °C eingefroren. Der aus dem enzymbehandelten Rohgut [1] gewonnene Saft wurde 2 min bei 98 °C zur Inaktivierung des Enzyms erhitzt und nach seinem schnellen Abkühlen unter den oben angegebenen Bedingungen eingefroren.

Saft aus roten Rüben, erhalten nach dem Pressen des gemahlenen Gutes [1] und nach Inaktivierung der Enzyme durch 2 min Erhitzen auf 98 °C, wurde bei −18 °C eingefroren.

Himbeeren wurden in Kartons von 500 g unter den oben erwähnten Bedingungen eingefroren.

Spinatpüree wurde durch Blanchieren des Rohgutes nach zwei Arten behandelt: a) 10−12 min in Wasser von 70 °C; b) 4−5 min mit Dampf. Nach dieser Behandlung wurde der Spinat passiert, schnell abgekühlt (Wasser- und Salzkühler) und portionsweise in paraffinierte Kartons von 600 g gegeben. Dort erfolgte das Gefrieren bei −18 °C innerhalb von 3,5 h.

Sellerie und Blumenkohl. Die Sellerie und der Blumenkohl wurden in etwa 1 cm große Schnitzel zerkleinert, 4 min in 0,1% Citronensäure enthaltendem siedendem Wasser blanchiert, mit fließendem Wasser abgekühlt und in Portionen von 1 kg bei −18 °C innerhalb von 4−4,5 h eingefroren.

Die gefrorenen pflanzlichen Produkte wurden 12 Monate in Gefrierräumen bei −18 °C und einer relativen Luftfeuchtigkeit von 95−98% aufbewahrt. Der MMS^+-Gehalt wurde jeden zweiten Monat durch eine Ionenaustauschreinigung und zweidimensionale Dünnschichtchromatographie [2] bestimmt.

Ergebnisse und Diskussion

Beim Verfolgen der Beständigkeit des MMS^+ in 0,02 M Citrat-Phosphat-Pufferlösungen mit pH 4,0, 6,0 und 8,0 sowie in Säften aus Sellerie mit pH 4,0 und aus roten Rüben mit pH 6,1 während 12 Monaten (Ampullen) wurde festgestellt, daß MMS^+ in der untersuchten Periode völlig stabil bleibt (Tab. 1).

Tabelle 1
Beständigkeit von MMS^+ in 0,02 M Citrat-Phosphat-Pufferlösungen und Pflanzensäften in % bei niedrigen Temperaturen während 12 Monaten

Art, pH und Konzentration der MMS^+-Lösungen	Beständigkeit [%]		
	+2 °C	−13 °C	−18 °C
I. *0,02 M Citrat-Phosphat-Pufferlösungen mit 20 µg MMS^+/cm^3*			
1. pH 4,0	100,0	101,0	100,0
2. pH 6,0	98,2	102,4	96,5
3. pH 8,0	95,0	98,0	97,4
II. *Pflanzensäfte*			
1. Saft aus Sellerie mit 60,5 µg MMS^+/cm^3 und pH 4,0	99,5	100,0	101,2
2. Saft aus roten Rüben mit 41,0 µg MMS^+/cm^3 und pH 6,1	98,3	99,1	100,0

Die Proben wurden in Ampullen aufbewahrt

Die Ergebnisse über den Gehalt an MMS^+ in frischen Pflanzensäften aus Sellerie und roten Rüben, Himbeeren, Blumenkohl und Spinatpüree und den daraus erhaltenen gefrorenen Proben zeigen, daß beim Gefrieren auf −18 °C während 3−5 h MMS^+ vollständig erhalten bleibt.

Beim Aufbewahren der auf diese Weise konservierten Produkte bei −18 °C werden im Verlauf von 12 Monaten keine wesentlichen Veränderungen im MMS^+-Gehalt beobachtet (Abb. 1). Seine Verluste erreichen im Sellerie- und Rote-Rüben-Saft am Ende des 12. Monats 10,6 bis 14,8%, und bei den Himbeeren überschreiten sie nicht 15,6%.

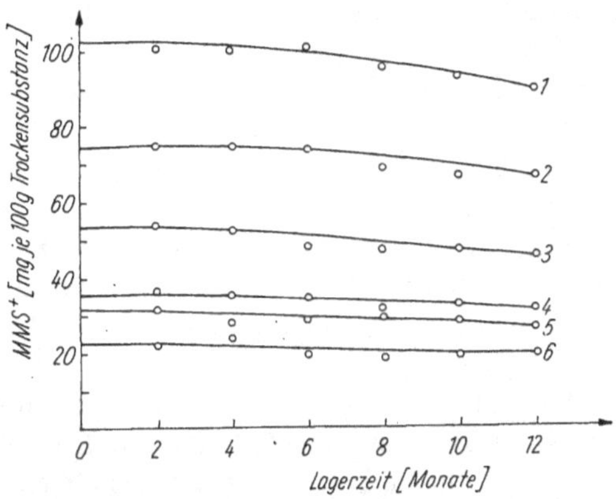

Abb. 1. Veränderung des MMS+-Gehaltes beim Aufbewahren von gefrorenen Produkten während 12 Monaten

1. Saft aus Sellerie, erhalten nach einer enzymatischen Behandlung des Rohgutes; 2. Saft aus Sellerie, erhalten nach einer thermischen Behandlung des Rohgutes; 3. Saft aus roten Rüben; 4. Himbeeren; 5. Blumenkohl; 6. Spinatpüree

Der beträchtlich niedrigere MMS+-Gehalt in den gefrorenen Halbfabrikaten aus Sellerie und Blumenkohl im Vergleich mit dem des Ausgangsrohgutes ist hauptsächlich auf die MMS+-Diffusion in das Wasser während des Blanchierens der Produkte vor dem Gefrieren zurückzuführen (Tab. 2). Bei der Sellerie gehen 23,9% und beim Blumenkohl 21,9% der ursprünglichen MMS+-Menge in die Wasserphase über. Die auf seinen Abbau bei der thermischen Behandlung während 4 min bei 98 °C zurückzuführenden Verluste betragen für Sellerie 11,6% und für Blumenkohl 10,2%, bezogen auf die Anfangsmenge an MMS+. Die Gesamtverluste an MMS+ beim Blanchieren

Tabelle 2
Beständigkeit von MMS+ beim Blanchieren von Spinat, Sellerie und Blumenkohl

Produkt und Blanchierbedingungen	MMS+-Gehalt						
	Im frischen Produkt			Im blanchierten Produkt			In Wasser
	Trockensubstanz [%]	[mg je 100 g Rohprodukt]	[mg je 100 g Trockensubstanz]	Trockensubstanz [%]	[mg je 100 g Rohprodukt]	[mg je 100 g Trockensubstanz]	in Wasser übergegangen [mg]
1. Spinat, 4–5 min mit Dampf behandelt	9,0	2,2	22,4	8,7	2,0	23,0	—
2. Spinat, 10–12 min in Wasser von 70 °C	9,0	2,2	22,4	7,4	1,4	18,9	1,9
3. Sellerie, 4 min in siedendem Wasser	11,0	5,8	52,7	10,6	3,6	34,0	12,6
4. Blumenkohl, 4 min in siedendem Wasser	10,6	5,0	47,1	10,0	3,2	32,0	10,3

von Sellerie und Blumenkohl im siedenden Wasserbad während 4 min betragen 35,5 bzw. 32,1%.

Mit der Diffusion von MMS^+ in die Wasserphase sind auch Verluste von 15,6% beim Wasserblanchieren des Spinats während 12 min bei 65—70 °C zu erklären, wogegen beim Behandeln von Spinatpüree mit Dampf während 4—5 min keine Verluste auftreten. Die Dampfbehandlung hat sich auch in der Industrie als bequemes und schnelles Verfahren zum Blanchieren von Spinatpüree durchgesetzt.

Bei der Aufbewahrung von gefrorenem Blumenkohl und Spinatpüree während 12 Monaten bei —18 °C wurden 15,6% Verlust an MMS^+ im Blumenkohl und 15,2% im Spinatpüree festgestellt (Abb. 1).

Aus den durchgeführten Versuchen kann die Schlußfolgerung gezogen werden, daß das geeignetste Konservierungsverfahren für pflanzliche Produkte deren Gefrieren bei niedrigen Temperaturen (—18 °C und darunter) ist. Nach einjährigem Aufbewahren der gefrorenen Naturprodukte bleiben 85 bis 90% des im Rohgut enthaltenen MMS^+ erhalten.

Summary

E. G. KOVATSCHEVA: Stability of S-methylmethionine in buffer solutions and vegetable products during their freezing conservation

The stability of S-methylmethionine (MMS^+) in citrate-phosphate buffer solutions (pH 4,0, 6,0, and 8,0) and juices of celery and beetroots (in ampullas) was investigated during twelve months with temperatures of +2, —13 and —18 °C. Besides, there was observed its stability during freezing and storage of its vegetable origins as celery, cauliflower, raspberry etc. in frozen state at a temperature of —18 °C. On the base of the results obtained we are in a position to recommend freezing conservation as the most suitable method for a maximum preservation of MMS^+ in its vegetable origins.

Резюме

Е. Г. Ковачева: устойчивость S — метилметионина в буферных растворах и растительных продуктах при их консервировании замораживанием

Исследована устойчивость S — Метилметионина (MMS^+) в цитратно-фосфатных буферных растворах с pH 4,00, 6,00 и 8,00 и в растительных соках из сельдеря и салатной свеклы (в ампулах) в течение 12 месяцев при +2, —13 и —18 °C. Кроме этого прослежена и его устойчивость при замораживании и сохранении в замороженном состоянии его растительных источников сельдеря, цветной капусты, малины и др. при температуре —18 °C.

На основании полученных результатов, рекомендуем применение метода консервирования замораживанием при низких температурах, как наиболее подходящий для максимального сохранения MMS^+ в его растительных источниках.

Literatur

[1] KOVATSCHEVA, E. G., Nahrung **22**, 315 (1978).
[2] KOVATSCHEVA, E. G., Nahrung **22**, 323 (1978).
[3] Sbornik technologitschni instrukzii za proizvodstvo na plodovi i zelentschukovi konservi. t. 2, DSO „Bulgarplod", Sofia (1971).

ELENA G. KOVATSCHEVA, Hochschule für Lebensmittelindustrie, Plovdiv, Boul. Lenin 26, VR Bulgarien

Eingegangen 2. 9. 1977

Die Nahrung	22	3	1978	335–345

Bezirks-Hygiene-Institut Karl-Marx-Stadt, (Direktor: Doz. Dr. sc. med. F. HAJDUK), Abteilung Lufthygiene, und Sektion Forstwirtschaft Tharandt der Technischen Universität Dresden, Wissenschaftsbereich Pflanzenchemie (Sektionsdirektor: Prof. Dr. sc. H. KURTH), DDR

Bewertung des Cadmiumgehaltes im Sedimentations- und Schwebstaub als Faktoren der Kontamination der Biosphäre

E. AUERMANN, H.-G. DÄSSLER, K. KÜNZEL, J. JACOBI und M. KNEUER

Auf einem Territorium von 3500 km^2 wurde an 63 Meßstellen in 52 Städten und Gemeinden der Cd-Ausfall aus der Atmosphäre im Durchschnitt zu 0,13–0,15 $mg/m^2 \cdot 30$ d bestimmt, während im Bereich schwermetallemittierender Industrie $\bar{x} = 0{,}33$ $mg/m^2 \cdot 30$ d beträgt. Im Aerosol liegt der Cd-Gehalt zwischen $\bar{x} = 0{,}003$ und 0,004 $\mu g\ m^{-3}$ bzw. 0,016 $\mu g\ m^{-3}$ bei Cd-emittierender Industrie. Der mittlere Anteil des Cadmiums am Sedimentationsstaub wurde zu 13–36 ppm errechnet. Die Cd-Belastung, gemessen als Cd-Niederschlag, korreliert mit der Größe des Siedlungsgebietes.
Als vorläufiger hygienisch noch zulässiger Schwellenwert werden im Aerosol 0,05 $\mu g\ m^{-3}$ und im Sedimentationsstaub 0,15 $mg/m^2 \cdot 30$ d empfohlen. Der Cd-Anteil im Sedimentationsstaub kann als eine ständige Belastung über die Nahrungskette angesehen werden, während vergleichsweise die Werte im Aerosol von untergeordneter Bedeutung für die Gesamtaufnahme des Menschen sind. Die pulmonale tägliche Aufnahme errechnet sich zu 0,075 μg; daraus kann die Resorption zu 0,038 μg eingeschätzt werden.

Der in den letzten Jahrzehnten beobachtete permanente Anstieg von Schadstoffen in der Luft, im Wasser und im Boden hat auch das Cadmium in den Blickpunkt gesundheitspolitischer Interessen rücken lassen. Nachweisbare Mengen in Pflanzen und in tierischen und menschlichen Organen mit teilweise bedenklichen Anreicherungen machen die Überwachung des Cadmiumgehaltes im Aerosol und im sedimentierbaren Staub erforderlich und dies nicht zuletzt, um Einfluß auf die Begrenzung der Emissionen zu nehmen oder Maßnahmen struktureller Natur in stark kontaminierten Bereichen anzustreben. Die vorliegende Arbeit soll die Kenntnisse über den Grad der Belastung des Territoriums erweitern und mögliche Zusammenhänge und Gesetzmäßigkeiten erkennen lassen.

Literaturübersicht

Emissionsquellen

Seit seiner Entdeckung durch STROMEYER (1817) ist Cadmium als Begleitkomponente von Zink, Kupfer und Blei in deren Erzen bekannt. Als Rohstoff für die Cadmiumerzeugung kommen vorrangig Flugstäube aus der Verhüttung dieser Erze in Betracht. Dagegen haben selbst Mineralien mit hohem Cadmiumgehalt infolge des geringen Umfanges ihres Vorkommens für eine technische Gewinnung keine Bedeutung.

Die breite Anwendung von Cadmium (Tab. 1) führt zu nur schwer beherrschbaren Verunreinigungsquellen. Neben den Emissionen der Hütten- und Verarbeitungsindustrie sind die Cadmiumgehalte

Tabelle 1
Haupteinsatzbereiche von Cadmium und seinen Verbindungen in der Industrie

Bestandteil niedrig schmelzende Legierungen wie
Woodsches Metall (12,5% Cd)
Lipowitzsches Metall (10% Cd)

Werkstoff für Lagermetalle (Legierung mit Ni, Cu)
Werkstoff für elektrische Kontakte (Legierung mit Ag, 20% Cd)
Werkstoff für Hartlot (5% Cd)
Werkstoff für Akkumulatorenbau (Ni-Cd-Sammler)

Oberflächenveredlung von Metallen (Galvanisieren, Elektroplattieren, Aufdampfen)

Verwendung in der Elektronik (Kathodenstrahlröhren, Selenzellen, Halbleiter etc.)
Verwendung in der Atomkernspaltung (Neutronenfänger)
Verwendung in der Photographie

Farbenherstellung
Stabilisatoren und Pigmente für die Kunststoffindustrie
Katalysator für chemische Prozesse
Reduktionsmittel
Herstellung von Imprägniermitteln
Herstellung von Pflanzen- und Holzschutzmitteln

in Stäuben aus kohle- und ölgefeuerten Heizungsanlagen (Tab. 2) nicht zu vernachlässigen. In Reingasstäuben aus Kraftwerken wurden durchschnittlich ca. 40 ppm Cd (maximal 115 ppm) nachgewiesen [1]. Am Ausgang der elektrischen Gasreinigungsanlage (EGR) eines Kohlekraftwerkes betrug die Cd-Konzentration 0,1 $\mu g\ m^{-3}$ [2]. Steinkohlenfeinstäube einer Kokerei enthielten 5—10 μg Cd g^{-1} Staub [3]. Schließlich ist Cadmium auch Bestandteil von Kraftfahrzeugabgasen.

Emissionsprobleme treten weiterhin bei der Altmetallaufbereitung, der Vernichtung von Kunststoffen in Müllverbrennungsanlagen, der Verregnung von Abwässern und der Ausbringung von Düngemitteln auf. Phosphordüngemittel enthalten beispielsweise bis zu 170 ppm Cd [4]. Während die Industrie- und die Kfz-Emissionen vor allem in begrenzten Territorien zu erhöhten Konzentrationen führen, bewirkt der Schadstoffauswurf von Heizwerken zunehmend eine großflächige Verunreinigung des Territoriums. Andererseits sind einer Steigerung der Cadmiumproduktion objektive Grenzen gesetzt. Das derzeit erreichte Verhältnis der Cadmium- zur Zinkgewinnung von 3 : 1000 ist kaum noch zu erhöhen, so daß bei dem wachsenden Bedarf dem Recycling dort, wo dafür technische Möglichkeiten gegeben sind (z. B. bei bestimmten Produktionsabwässern), sowohl im Interesse des Umwelt-

Tabelle 2
Cadmium in Brenn- und Kraftstoffen, Kohlenstäuben und -aschen

Material	Cadmiumgehalt	Literatur
Kohle	1—2 ppm	[5]
Dieselöl	$\leqq$ 0,53 ppm	[5]
Benzin	10—35 ppb	[6]
Heizöl	0,42—0,53 ppm	[5]
Kohlenstaub		[3]
— Steinkohlenaufbereitung	5 ppm	
— Koksofenbatterie	9 ppm	
— Kokssortierung	10 ppm	
Reingasstaub		[1]
(20 Proben aus Kohlekraftwerken)	im Mittel 40 ppm maximal 115 ppm	
Staub am Filterausgang eines Kohlekraftwerkes (EGR)	0,1 $\mu g\ m^{-3}$	[2]

schutzes als auch zugunsten der Materialökonomie, große Bedeutung zukommt. Die breite Palette der industriellen Anwendung von Cd offenbart neben seiner wirtschaftlichen Bedeutung zugleich die Schwierigkeiten bei einer ökonomisch vertretbaren Rückgewinnung des Schwermetalls. Die Recyclingrate in der BRD beträgt z. Z. 5% [7].

Cadmiumgehalt der Luft

Schätzungsweise liegt die Cadmiumemission bei einem Drittel der Cadmiumproduktion [8]. Allein bei einem Kohlekraftwerk mit einer Kapazität von 1200 MW ist mit ca. 17—34 kg Cadmium pro Jahr im Auswurf bzw. Rückstand zu rechnen [3]. Bei der Gewinnung von Cadmium durch Destillation betragen die Verdampfungsverluste bis zu 49% [10].

Die Gefährlichkeit cadmiumhaltiger Abgase und Stäube hat sich am Beispiel großer Nebelkatastrophen offenbart. Im Jahre 1948 erkrankten in Donora (Pennsylvania, USA) im Verlaufe einer Inversionswetterlage 5910 Personen. Die Emissionen entstammten der Stahl- und Zinkhüttenindustrie [11]. Der Cadmiumanteil in der Luft sollte jedoch nicht isoliert gesehen werden. Wesentliche Bedeutung kommt sicher der komplexen Wirkung verschiedener Schadfaktoren zu.

Die bei der Verbrennung von Kohle in Kraftwerken entstehenden Staubteilchen weisen den höchsten Gehalt an toxischen Spurenelementen, inbegriffen Cadmium, im lungengängigen Korngrößenbereich, also unter 5 µm, auf [12]. Diese feinen Staubteilchen haben in der Atmosphäre eine Verweilzeit bis zu einigen Jahren und dadurch bedingt auch eine große Reichweite. Die Grundbelastung der atmosphärischen Luft liegt generell unter 0,001 µg Cd m^{-3}. In Großstädten können Monats- und Jahresmittelwerte bis zu 0,05 µg Cd m^{-3} erreichen. In der Umgebung von Cadmiumemittenten kommen Wochen- und Monatsmittel bis zu 0,3 µg Cd m^{-3} vor [13]. Konzentrationen von mehr als 1 µg Cd m^{-3} sind auch in der Nähe von Cadmiumproduzenten selten [14]. Eine Zusammenstellung in der Literatur angegebener Meßwerte enthält Tab. 3.

Die 1. DB zur 5. Durchführungsverordnung zum Landeskulturgesetz „Reinhaltung der Luft" [30] gibt für Cadmium noch keine Immissionsgrenzwerte (MIK-Werte) an. Das International Hearing des VDI der BRD (1973) gab die Empfehlung, eine maximale Konzentration von 0,05 µg Cd m^{-3} Luft als Grenzwert festzusetzen. Aussagen über eine Dosis zur Verhinderung von Langzeiteffekten können gegenwärtig nicht getroffen werden. Viele Autoren befürworten als hygienisch zulässigen MAK-Wert 0,1 mg Cd m^{-3}. Die tägliche Aufnahme von Cadmium mit der Atemluft beträgt ca. 0,02 µg in unbelasteten Gebieten, ca. 1 µg in Großstädten und ca. 4—12 µg in der Nähe von Cadmiumemittenten (Atemvolumen des Menschen: 20 m^3 d^{-1}). Davon unterliegen etwa 10 bis 40% der Resorption [22].

Tabelle 3
Cadmium [µg m^{-3}] in der atmosphärischen Luft

Meßort	Immissionsmeßwert	Literatur
Frankfurt/M., Innenstadt	0,06	[15]
Frankfurt/M, Wohngebiet	0,03	[15]
Gelsenkirchen/Industriegebiet	0,01—0,145	[16]
Schauinsland/Schwarzwald	0,0001—0,001	[16]
Mainz	$\bar{x}$ = 0,0015 März 1972 0,010 Januar 1972 0,004	[16]
verkehrs- und industrieferne Gebiete	0,005—0,009	[15]
500—100 m entfernt von einem Cd-Emittent	0,2—0,6	[6]
Mittelwert in amerikanischen Städten	0,002	[17]
Maximum in amerikanischen Städten	0,420	
Raum Stockholm, Wochendurchschnitt	0,005	[18]
Raum Erlangen, Wochendurchschnitt	0,0015	[19]
Schwedisches Industriegebiet	0,3—0,6	[18]
Japanisches Industriegebiet	0,1—0,3	[20]
Autotunnel	0,9	[21]

Zur Toxizität des Cadmiums

Der Organismus besitzt gegenüber Schwermetallen ein hohes Kompensationsvermögen [23]. Eingehende Untersuchungen von FRIBERG u. a. [18], die auf Veranlassung des US Department of Health durchgeführt worden sind, haben das Ergebnis erbracht, daß bisher nachgewiesene chronische Vergiftungen durch Umwelt-Cadmium, wenn überhaupt, lediglich in Japan vorgekommen sind. Auch dort soll die Itai-Itai-Krankheit (rachitisähnliche Knochenveränderung) nur im Komplex mit anderen Schadfaktoren zu sehen gewesen sein, obwohl die Aufnahme in den stark kontaminierten Gebieten über 10 bis 20 Jahre hinweg etwa 600 μg Cd d^{-1} betragen hat [24]. Die Aufnahmerate in Europa liegt bei ca. 25 bis 75 μg d^{-1} [13].

Cadmium zählt zu den starken Giften. Seine Wirkung beruht maßgeblich auf Störungen im biochemischen und enzymatischen Bereich [23]. Wichtigstes Primärereignis im toxikologischen Sinne ist die Enzyminhibition und im weiteren Verlauf unter Bildung von Metallalbuminaten eine Denaturierung der Eiweißkörper. Die größte Gefährdung geht vom verdampfenden metallischen Cadmium aus. Es folgen Cadmiumoxid-Dämpfe und -Stäube, reiner Metallstaub und cadmiumhaltige Stäube [24, 25]. Äußerst giftig sind wasser- und säurelösliche Verbindungen.

Cadmium gilt als kanzerogen, nephrotoxisch und hypertensiv [9]. Im Vordergrund steht die Wirkung auf den Respirationstrakt [26]. In Leber und Niere von an Lungenemphysem und Karzinom Verstorbenen wurde signifikant mehr Cd gefunden als bei anderen Todesursachen [8]. Diese Organe gelten als bevorzugte Akkumulationsorte für Cadmium.

Im Zusammenhang mit der chronischen Wirkung von Cadmium werden von den meisten Autoren übereinstimmend folgende Symptome genannt: Anfänglichen unspezifischen Anzeichen wie Müdigkeit, Nervosität, Reizbarkeit, Durst, Husten, Nasenlaufen, Kurzatmigkeit und Magen-Darm-Störungen folgen

- Veränderungen in den Atemwegen bis zu Lungenemphysem
- Nieren- und Leberschädigung, Proteinurie
- Cadmiumschnupfen mit degenerativen Veränderungen im Nasen-Rachen-Raum bis zur Geschwürbildung
- Cadmiumsaum am Zahnhals
- Anämie
- Chronische Bronchitis (ohne nachweisbares Emphysem)
- Knochenveränderungen im Sinne von Skelettschäden.

Bis zum Eintreten erster subjektiver und objektiver Erscheinungen kann eine Latenzzeit von mehreren Jahren vergehen.

Eigene Untersuchungen

Probeentnahme

Zur Ermittlung des Cadmiumgehaltes der Luft erfolgte dessen Bestimmung im Schweb- und Sedimentationsstaub. Die Beschränkung der Untersuchungen auf Schwebstaub halten wir für unzureichend. Dieser dient zwar der Einschätzung der Cd-Aufnahme des Menschen über den Atemtrakt, Sedimentationsstäube jedoch charakterisieren eindeutig die Belastung des Territoriums und geben Hinweise über den Grad der Kontamination von Pflanzen, Trinkwasser, Boden und somit über die Aufnahme in die Nahrungskette. Durch Agglomerationsvorgänge kann eine Abreicherung des Schwebstaubgehaltes eintreten und somit die Belastung der Territorien aerosolseitig unterschiedlich ausweisen.

Über ein Territorium von 3500 km² wurden in 52 Städten und Gemeinden 63 Meßpunkte verteilt. Das so erhaltene Meßnetz weist Gebiete mit großstädtischem Charakter, mittlere Städte, Kleinstädte, Gemeinden im ländlichen Bereich und unbewohnte Gegenden aus. Lokale Einflüsse wurden durch die Lage der Meßpunkte ausgeschaltet. Die Meßergebnisse repräsentieren somit eine durchschnittliche Schadstoffbelastung der jeweiligen Siedlungsgebiete. Die Proben wurden nach einem festgelegten Ablaufplan turnusgemäß in den Jahren 1975—1976 entnommen.

Untersuchungsmethode

1. Probenahme und Aufschluß der Proben

Für die Abscheidung des Schwebstaubes dienten Membranfilter Synpor 4 (∅ 35 mm, mittlere Porengröße 0,85 μm) der Firma Synthesia (ČSSR), die in Schraubkasetten auf Metallsinterplatten eingelegt wurden, wobei sich das durchgesaugte Luftvolumen zwischen 3 und 4 m^3 bewegte. Zur Ermittlung der Staubmenge werden die vortarierten Filter unter reproduzierbaren Bedingungen ausgewogen und zwecks atomabsorptionsspektrometrischer Cadmium-Bestimmung in 10 ml konz. Salpetersäure durch Aufkochen gelöst. Nach dem Einengen auf etwa 1 ml wird die Probe mit 5 ml bidest. Wasser versetzt, aufgekocht und auf 10 ml aufgefüllt.

Der Aufschluß der in Staubsammelgefäßen gezogenen Sedimentationsstaubproben (Expositionsdauer: 30 d) erfolgte nach der Auswaage der Gesamtstaubmenge durch Aufkochen mit 10 ml konz. Salzsäure, zu der man vorsichtig 2 ml konz. Salpetersäure tropfen läßt. Unter vollständigem Vertreiben der nitrosen Gase engt man auf 3—4 ml ein, gibt 15 ml bidest. Wasser hinzu und filtriert durch ein mit Säure gewaschenes Filter in einen 25-ml-Meßkolben. Das Filter wird mit 0,1 N Salzsäure nachgewaschen und der Meßkolben bis zur Eichmarke aufgefüllt. In den so vorbereiteten Lösungen können neben Cadmium weitere Metalle bestimmt werden.

2. Atomabsorptionsspektrometrische Bestimmungen

Die Cd-Bestimmungen erfolgten nach der flammenlosen Methode mit dem AAS-Gerät 300 S von Perkin-Elmer unter Verwendung eines Deuteriumuntergrundkompensators und der Graphitrohrküvette HGA 72 als Zusatzgerät.

Folgende Parameter wurden für die Analysen gewählt:

Wellenlänge: 228,8 nm
Spektrale Spaltbreite: 0,7 nm
Lampenstrom: 8 mA
Programm 1 30 s bei 96 °C (Trocknen)
Programm 2 30 s bei 320 °C (Zersetzen)
Programm 3 10 s bei 1800 °C (Atomisieren)
Programm 4 10 s bei 2600 °C (Ausglühen)

Spülgas: Argon
Skalendehnung: 3
Probenvolumen: 20 μl

Für die Auswertung der Proben mußte auf Grund der unterschiedlichen Matrices die Additionsmethode angewendet werden. Zu ihrer Durchführung wurden von der Probe 4 aliquote Teile entnommen und 3 dieser Anteile das gleiche Volumen einer Eichlösung verschiedener Konzentration zugesetzt. Die vierte Probe wird mit dem gleichen Volumen dest. Wasser verdünnt. Durch Auftragen der Peakhöhen der Proben gegen die zugesetzte Cadmiummenge erhält man eine Gerade, die die Extinktionsachse in einem Punkt schneidet, der dem Cadmiumgehalt der Probe entspricht. Durch Extrapolation der Extinktionswerte gegen Null bekommt man die Cadmiumkonzentration der betreffenden Probelösung.

Im Falle der Schwebstaubproben ist es möglich, die Auswertung dahingehend zu vereinfachen, daß man aus der oben beschriebenen Eichkurve durch Parallelverschiebung eine Ausgleichsgerade zeichnet, die durch den Nullpunkt läuft. Mit Hilfe dieser Ausgleichsgeraden können alle folgenden Schwebstaubproben bestimmt werden [28]. Voraussetzung für die Auswertung der Additionsmethode ist, daß alle Messungen in linearem Bereich liegen.

Die Nachweisgrenze [29], berechnet aus dem Mittel der Blindwerte der Aufschlußlösungen und ihrer dreifachen Standardabweichung, ergab für Schwebstaubproben 0,0003 μg Cd ml^{-1} und für Sedimentationsstaubproben 0,0008 μg Cd ml^{-1}. Für Schwebstaub ergibt sich damit bei einem Luftdurchsatz von 3 m^3 und einem Probevolumen von 10 ml eine relative Nachweisgrenze von 0,001 μg Cd m^{-3} und für Sedimentationsstaub von 0,02 μg Cd/Probe bzw. bei 30 Tagen Expositionszeit nach der Weckglasmethode 3,3 μg Cd/m^2 · 30 d.

Ergebnisse

Zur Prüfung der Abhängigkeit der Cd-Konzentrationen von der Größe und dem industriellen Charakter des Siedlungsgebietes erfolgte eine Aufgliederung der Ergebnisse für die einzelnen Meßstellen gemäß nachstehender Gliederung:

1. Unbewohntes Gebiet
2. Siedlungen mit 1000—10000 Einwohner
3. Siedlungen mit 10000—100000 Einwohner
4. Siedlungen größer als 100000 Einwohner
5. Siedlungen mit Schwermetallindustrie

Bei den Gruppen 2—4 wurden die Siedlungen mit schwermetallemittierender Industrie herausgenommen. Die Gruppe 1 repräsentiert die Kammlagen des Erzgebirges, welche unter der Fernwirkung der Emissionen der sächsischen und nordböhmischen Industrie stehen.

In Abb. 1 ist die relative Summenhäufigkeitsverteilung des sedimentierenden Cadmiumanteils der Meßwerte für die Gruppen 1—5 dargestellt. Hierbei zeigt sich, daß die Ausgleichsgeraden für die Gebiete 1—4 in einem sehr engen Bereich zusammenliegen. Von diesem hebt sich deutlich die Ausgleichsgerade für die Siedlungsgebiete mit Schwermetallindustrie ab. Außerdem deutet sich eine ansteigende Belastung in den Gruppen 2—4 an. Die Belastung in den Kammlagen ordnet sich zwischen den Gruppen 2 und 3 ein. Zur Klärung, inwieweit sich die Verteilungen in den Gruppen 1—5 signifikant unterscheiden, wurden diese, bei einer Irrtumswahrscheinlichkeit von 1%, nach Kolmogorov-Smirnov getestet. Nach den Testergebnissen weichen die Territorien der Schwermetallindustrie bezüglich ihrer Verteilung von allen anderen Gebieten (1—4) signifikant ab. Signifikante Unterschiede bestehen auch zwischen den Gruppen 4 und 2, d. h. die Gruppe 2 ist bezgl. Cadmium im Sedimentationsstaub als geringer belastet zu bewerten. Alle anderen Gruppen sind nach den vorläufigen Ergebnissen als gleichartig zu betrachten. Die Fortführung der Untersuchungen zur weiteren Absicherung der Ergebnisse erscheint nach den mathematischen Betrachtungen sinnvoll. Bei Vergrößerung der Probenzahl kann es gelingen, weitere signifikante Unterschiede nachzuweisen.

In Abb. 2 sind die Ausgleichsgeraden für folgende Gruppeneinteilung dargestellt:

A Gesamtheit aller Meßstellen
B Gesamtheit aller Meßstellen mit Ausschluß von C
C Gesamtheit der Meßstellen mit Schwermetallbelastung.

Die Lage und der Anstieg der Kurve B weisen das zugehörige Gebiet als am geringsten belastet aus.

In Tab. 4 sind die abzuleitenden Parameter aufgeführt. Danach beträgt die durchschnittliche Cd-Belastung für Gebiete ohne schwermetallemittierende Industrie 0,13 $mg/m^2 \cdot 30$ d. Die Einzelwerte liegen zwischen 0,01 und 0,47 $mg/m^2 \cdot 30$ d. Im Bereich der Schwermetallindustrie treten Maximalwerte bis 1 $mg/m^2 \cdot 30$ d auf.

Um weitere Informationen zu erhalten, erfolgte die Berechnung des massebezogenen Cd-Anteils im Sedimentationsstaub. Tab. 5 beinhaltet die Parameter der einzelnen Siedlungsgebiete. Zum besseren Vergleich wurden die Territorien nach steigenden Parameterwerten aufgelistet. Lediglich für die Spalte x_{max} ergab sich nicht die gleiche Rangfolge, eine Tatsache, die auch nicht von vornherein zu erwarten ist.

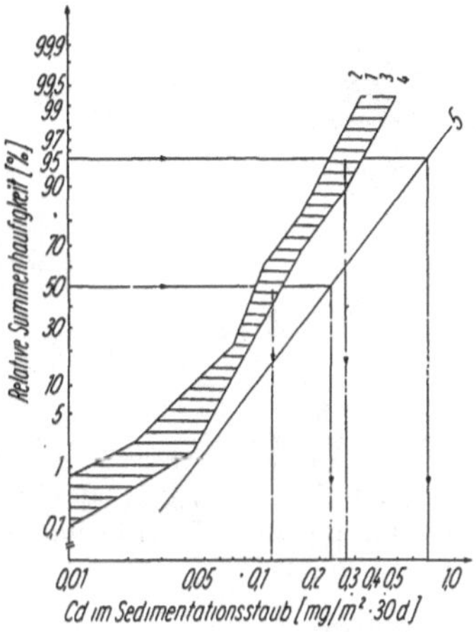

Abb. 1. Relative Summenhäufigkeitsverteilung des sedimentierenden Cadmiums für die Gebiete 1 bis 5

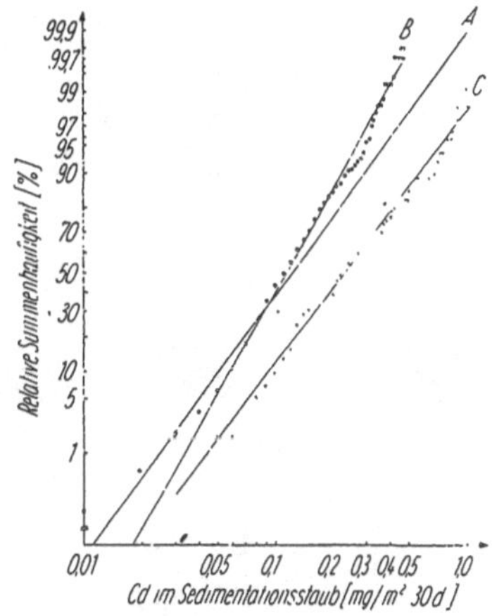

Abb. 2. Relative Summenhäufigkeitsverteilung des sedimentierenden Cadmiums für die Gebiete A, B und C

Tabelle 4
Mittelwerte, Standardabweichungen, 50%- und 95%-Werte von Cadmium [$mg/m^2 \cdot 30$ d] im Sedimentationsstaub der Territorien A, B und C

Gruppe	Arithmetischer Mittelwert $\bar{x}$	Standardabweichung s	50%-Wert	95%-Wert
A	0,155	0,196	0,123	0,375
B	0,132	0,073	0,115	0,270
C	0,328	0,398	0,230	0,730

Tabelle 5
Massebezogener Anteil des Cadmiums [ppm] im Sedimentationsstaub aus den Siedlungsgebieten 1–5

Gebiet	arithmetischer Mittelwert $\bar{x}$	Standard-abweichung s	Variabilitäts-koeffizient V [%]	maximaler Einzelwert x_{max}	50%-Wert x	95%-Wert
4	12,6	9,2	73	47	10,0	31,5
3	14,6	10,9	75	94	11,8	33,2
2	15,9	12,0	76	63	12,4	40,0
1	30,7	29,3	96	147	20,6	94,0
5	36,5	52,8	145	433	22,2	100,4
Gesamtheit aller Meß-stellen (1–5)	22,0	28,3	129	433	14,1	60,0

Nach Prüfung der relativen Summenhäufigkeitsverteilungen (Abb. 3) mit Hilfe des Kolmogorov-Smirnov-Testes sind bei einer Irrtumswahrscheinlichkeit von 1% die Gruppen 2–4 als gleich einzustufen. Das gleiche gilt für die Gruppen 1 und 5. Hinsichtlich ihrer Verteilung unterscheiden sich jeweils die Bereiche 1 und 5 gegenüber denen von 2–4.

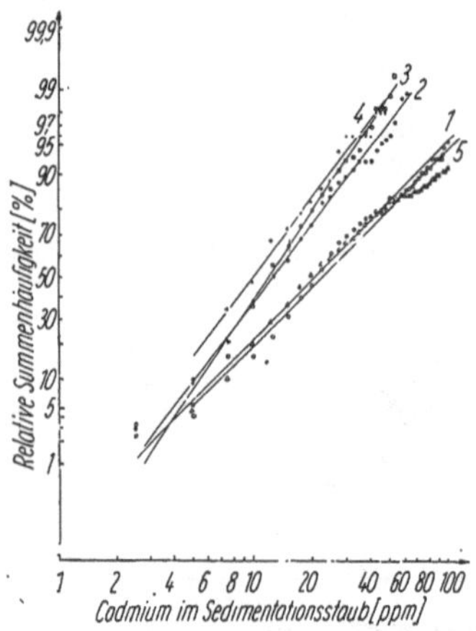

Abb. 3. Relative Summenhäufigkeitsverteilung des massebezogenen Anteils des Cadmiums im Sedimentationsstaub

Tab. 6 enthält die Kenngrößen des Cd-Gehaltes im Schwebstaub. Die Werte bewegen sich bei Ausschluß der Cd-Emittenten zwischen 0,001 und 0,012 $\mu g\ m^{-3}$. Die durchschnittliche Konzentration beträgt hier 0,004 $\mu g\ m^{-3}$. In den Territorien mit Cd-emittierender Industrie konnten Maximalwerte bis 0,060 und 0,070 $\mu g\ m^{-3}$ erfaßt werden; die zugehörige durchschnittliche Konzentration liegt bei 0,016 $\mu g\ m^{-3}$.

Der massebezogene Anteil des Cadmiums im Schwebstaub für die Gebiete 2–5 beläuft sich im Durchschnitt auf 47 ppm mit einer Variationsbreite von 1–167 ppm (Tab. 7). Für die Kammlage des Erzgebirges (Gebiet 1) wurden Werte zwischen 21 und 194 ppm mit $\bar{x} = 74$ ppm ermittelt.

Tabelle 6
Mittelwerte, Standardabweichung und maximale Einzelwerte von Cadmium [$\mu g\ m^{-3}$] im Schwebstaub aus den Siedlungsgebieten 1–5

Gebiet	arithmetischer Mittelwert $\bar{x}$	Standardabweichung s	maximaler Einzelwert x_{max}
1	0,003	0,001	0,012
2–4	0,004	0,001	0,009
5	0,016	0,028	0,070
Gesamtheit aller Meßstellen (1–5)	0,005	0,012	0,070

Tabelle 7
Massebezogener Anteil des Cadmiums [ppm] im Schwebstaub aus den Siedlungsgebieten 1–5

Gebiet	arithmetischer Mittelwert $\bar{x}$	Standardabweichung s	maximaler Einzelwert x_{max}	Variabilitätskoeffizient V [%]
2–5	47	39	167	82
1	74	52	194	70

Diskussion

Die Ergebnisse der Studie lassen deutlich die Rohbraunkohle als Hauptquelle der Cd-Beaufschlagung des Territoriums erkennen. Diese Schlußfolgerung leitet sich zwingend aus Tab. 5 ab, nach der in den Siedlungsgebieten bei Eliminierung jener durch spezielle Cd-Emittenten belasteten Bereiche ein fast von der Größe des Siedlungsgebietes unabhängiger prozentualer Anteil Cadmium im Sedimentationsstaub enthalten ist. Da in der DDR die Hauptenergiequelle Rohbraunkohle darstellt, ist die relative massebezogene Gleichheit von Cd im Sedimentationsstaub verständlich. Gleichzeitig ist die Rohbraunkohle die bedeutendste Quelle der Staubbelastung. Abb. 1 zeigt den Anstieg der flächenbezogenen Beaufschlagung von Cd mit steigender Größe des Siedlungsgebietes, das wiederum allgemein mit der durch Verbrennungsanlagen hervorgerufenen Emissionsdichte der Heizungsanlagen korreliert. Erste Analysen der in einem Heizkraftwerk eingesetzten Rohbraunkohle (Zwenkauer Revier) zeigten einen Cd-Gehalt von 0,7 ppm im lufttrockenen Rohprodukt. In der Filterasche konnte 1 ppm bestimmt werden. Hierin liegt auch die ubiquitäre Verteilung des Cadmiums in der Atmosphäre begründet. Selbst in Gebieten mit ausgesprochen land- und forstwirtschaftlichem Charakter ist es nachweisbar. Verantwortlich für sein Auftreten weitab von der Emissionsquelle ist das Cd-haltige Aerosol. Der Cd-Anteil im Schwebestaub ist etwa um das 3fache höher als im Sedimentationsstaub. Durch Agglomeration des Aerosols tritt dieses Element auch weit entfernt von den industriellen Emissionsquellen im Sedimentationsstaub auf. Sicher ist an diesen Konzentrationen auch der natürliche Cd-Gehalt des Bodens beteiligt, der durch Erosion und Aufwirbelung zur sekundären Belastung der Atmosphäre führt. Weitere Untersuchungen zum Cd-Gehalt der Böden in dem Untersuchungsgebiet werden Aufschlüsse über den jeweiligen Anteil ergeben. Welche Überlegungen ergeben sich für die Belastung der Biosphäre? Mit einer durchschnittlichen Belastung von 0,13—0,16 mg/m^2 · 30d erfolgt eine ständige Cd-Zufuhr auf den Boden für die Pflanzen sowie auf die Oberflächengewässer und findet hierüber den Eingang in die Nahrungskette. Im Untersuchsgebiet mit einer Fläche von 3500 km^2 kann mit einer jährlichen Cd-Beaufschlagung von 5,5—6,7 t bzw. 1,56 bis 1,92 kg pro km^2 gerechnet werden.

Für die pulmonale Aufnahme des Menschen ist der Staub mit einer Korngröße $>$ 10 μm bedeutungslos. Für diese Betrachtung muß der Cd-Gehalt im Aerosol herangezogen werden. Legt man eine durchschnittliche Belastung von 0,005 μg m^{-3} (Tab. 6) zugrunde, so werden bei einem Atemvolumen von 15 m^3/24 h 0,075 μg Cadmium aufgenommen. Davon dürften etwa max. 50% in die Blutbahn gelangen, was einer pulmonalen täglichen Resorption von 0,038 μg entspricht. Damit dürfte der Cd-Gehalt im Aerosol für die Gesamtaufnahme des Menschen von untergeordneter Bedeutung sein. Dagegen sehen wir in der Kontamination der Nahrungsmittel (Gemüse, Obst, Getreideprodukte, Hackfrüchte, Futtermittel) durch cadmiumhaltige Sedimentationsstäube die ursächliche Quelle. Eine Betrachtung der in der internationalen Literatur zitierten Werte zeigte, daß die Belastung in unseren Wohngebieten im unteren Bereich vergleichbarer Industrieländer liegt. Die Angaben aus Japan, Schweden und der BRD sind teilweise um eine Zehnerstelle angehoben. Wenn über Cd-Anreicherungen in der Leber und Niere berichtet wird [27], so muß die Hauptaufnahme des Cadmiums über die Nahrungskette gesehen werden, wofür als Quelle, wie bereits dargelegt, der Anteil im Sedimentationsstaub zu sehen ist.

Für die operative Tätigkeit der Bezirks-Hygiene-Inspektion, z. B. bei der lufthygienischen Beurteilung von Investvorhaben, der Bearbeitung von Grenzwertbescheiden oder bei der Forderung nach Anlagen zur Luftreinhaltung, ist die Kenntnis des hygienisch zulässigen Schwellenwertes (MIK-Wert) erforderlich. Da die o. a. 5. Durchführungsverordnung zum Landeskulturgesetz noch keinen derartigen Grenzwert ausweist, empfehlen wir zur einheitlichen Beurteilung von Anlagen durch die Bezirks-Hygiene-Inspektion auf der Grundlage unseres Literaturstudiums sowie der erzielten und statistisch bearbeiteten Meßergebnisse als vorläufigen MIK-Wert im Aerosol 0,05 $\mu g\ m^{-3}$ und im Sedimentationsstaub als noch zulässigen Jahresmittelwert 0,15 $mg/m^2 \cdot 30d$.

Schlußfolgerungen

Der Cd-Gehalt des Aerosols ist mit Ausnahme im Bereich Cd-emittierender Industrie niedrig. Relevant sind die Konzentrationen im Sedimentationsstaub. Sie können im Territorium zu einer Belastung der Biosphäre und über die Nahrungskette zur erhöhten Speicherung in tierischen und menschlichen Organen führen. Durch verstärkten Einbau von Staubabscheidern in Heizungsanlagen kann dieser Belastung erfolgreich entgegengewirkt werden. Hierbei ist dem Einsatz von leistungsfähigen Entstaubungssystemen zur Abscheidung von Feinstäuben Beachtung zu schenken. Die in den letzten Jahren in der DDR eingeleiteten Maßnahmen zur Emissionsbegrenzung auf der Grundlage der 5. DVO zum Landeskulturgesetz müssen zielstrebig auch im Sinne der Absenkung der Cd-Belastung fortgeführt werden.

Summary

E. AUERMANN, H. G. DÄSSLER, K. KÜNZEL, J. JACOBI and M. KNEUER: Evaluation of the cadmium content in sedimentary and air-borne dusts as factors of the contamination of the biosphere

In a territory being 3.500 km^2, the cadmium deposits from the atmosphere were determined at 63 sites in 52 towns and communities. These determinations yielded a mean value ranging from 0.13 to 0.15 $mg/m^2 \cdot 30$ d. On the contrary, the mean value ($\bar{x}$) was 0.33 $mg/m^2 \cdot 30$ d in the region of heavy-metal-emitting industries. The mean cadmium content in the aerosol was between 0.003 and 0.004 $\mu g\ m^{-3}$ and, respectively, 0.016 $\mu g\ m^{-3}$ in case of cadmium emission. It was calculated that the mean proportion of cadmium in the sedimentary dust was between 13 and 16 p.p.m. The cadmium burden, as estimated as cadmium sediment, correlated with the extent of the developmental area.

The authors recommend for the present the following maximum permissible values: 0.05 $\mu g\ m^{-3}$ in the aerosol, and 0.15 $mg/m^2 \cdot 30$ d. The cadmium content in the sedimentary dust may be considered to be a permanent burden applied via the food chain, whereas the content in the aerosol is of less importance to the total uptake in man. The calculation of the daily pulmonary uptake yielded a value of 0.075 μg, from which an absorption of 0.038 μg is estimated.

Резюме

Е. Ауерманн, Х.-Г. Деслер, К. Кюнцель, Й. Якоби и М. Кнойер: Оценка содержания кадмия в витающей и седиментационной пыли как факторы загрязнения биосферы

На территории в 3500 км² в 52 городах и селах в 63 точках выпад кадмия из атмосферы составлял в среднем 0,13—0,15 $мг/м^2 \cdot 30$ d, в то время как областях тяжелой металлургии $\bar{x} = 0,33$ $мг/м^2$ 30 d. В аэрозоле содержание кадмия колебался от $\bar{x} = 0,003$ и 0,004 $мкг\ м^{-3}$ или 0,016 $мкг\ м^{-3}$ при наличии выделяющей кадмий промышленности. Среднее процентное содержание кадмия в седиментационной пыли по расчету составляет 13—36 ppm. Нагрузка кадмием, вытекающая из осаждения кадмия, коррелирует с величиной населенной местности.

В качестве гигиенически еще допустимой пороговой величины рекомендуются дляаэрозоли 0,05 мкг $м^{-3}$ и для седиментационной пыли 0,15 кмг/$м^2$ · 30 d. Содержание кадмия в седиментационной пыли является постоянной нагрузкой действуя через пищевую цепь, в то время как например данные аэрозоля не имеют существенного значения для общего поступления у человека. Легочное поступление за сутки определяется в 0,075 мкг; отсюда всасывание оценивается в 0,038 мкг.

Literatur

[1] Kautz, K., H. Kirsch u. D. W. Laufhütte, VGB Kraftwerkstechnik **55**, 672—676 (1975).

[2] Lee, R. E., H. L. Crist, A. E. Riley u. K. E. MacLeod, Environm. Sci. Technol. **9**, 643—647 (1975).

[3] Masek, V., Zbl. Arb.-Med. u. Arb.-Schutz **24**, 332—339 (1974).

[4] Kloke, A., Nachrichtenbl. dtsch. Pflanzenschutzdienst **23**, 164—167 (1971).

[5] Page, A. L., u. F. T. Bingham, zit. nach Gunther, F. A., u. J. D. Gunther, Residue reviews **48**, 1—44 (1973).

[6] Nordberg, G. F., Ambio **3**, 55—66 (1974).

[7] Teworte, W., Staub — Reinhalt. Luft **33**, 422—431 (1973).

[8] Anke, M., A. Hennig, H.-J. Schneider, B. Groppel, M. Grün, M. Partschefeld u. H. Lüdke, Wiss. Z. Karl-Marx-Univ. Leipzig, Math.-Naturwiss. R., **25**, 241—261 (1976).

[9] Schenkling, V., Nachrichten Mensch — Umwelt **3**, 1—31 (1975).

[10] Mielnikowa, E. A., Gig: i San. **22**, Heft 3, 25—31 (1957).

[11] Baader, E. W., Dtsch. med. Wschr. **75**, 513—516 (1950).

[12] Natusch, D. F. S., J. R. Wallace u. C. A. Evans, Science **183**, 202—204 (1974).

[13] Piscator, M., Staub — Reinhalt. Luft **33**, 457—459 (1973).

[14] Hartkamp, H., Staub — Reinhalt. Luft **34**, 12—15 (1974).

[15] Georgii, H. W., VDI-Berichte Nr. 203, 1974.

[16] Neeb, R., u. F. Wahdat, Z. Anal. Chem. 269, 275—279 (1974).

[17] Israel, H., u. G. W. Israel, Spurenstoffe in der Atmosphäre. Wissenschaftliche Verlagsgesellschaft, Stuttgart 1973.

[18] Friberg, L., M. Piscator u. G. Norberg, Cadmium in the environment, CRC-Press, Cleveland, Ohio, 1971.

[19] Larsson, J. E., Cadmium in man's environment. For the WHO regional Office for Europe, Copenhagen, Dänemark, 1973.

[20] WHO Techn. Rep. Ser. 505, 1—32 (1972).

[21] Tesarova, M., Chemické listy **68**, 12—22 (1974).

[22] Förstner, U., u. G. Müller, Schwermetalle in Flüssen und Seen. Springer-Verlag Berlin, Heidelberg, New York 1974.

[23] Hirth, L., Münchener med. Wochenschr. **106**, 985—988 (1964).

[24] Ullmanns Enzyklopädie der Technischen Chemie. 4. Aufl., Bd. 9, S. 58—61. Verlag Chemie, Weinheim/Bergstraße 1975.

[25] Fischer, H., Gewerbliche Vergiftungen durch Cadmium, Quecksilber, Arsen und ihre Verbindungen. Schriften der Gesellschaft Deutscher Metallhütten und Bergleute e. V., Heft 6. Clausthal Zellerfeld 1958.

[26] Kaffer, H. R., Das Krankheitsbild der gewerblichen Vergiftung durch Cadmium oder seine Verbindungen. Dissertation, Bonn 1961.

[27] Cumbrowski, J., u. W. Raffke, Z. ges. Hyg. **21**, 1—7 (1975).

[28] Fleischer, M., Perkin-Almer Analysen — technische Berichte, Heft 33.

[29] Kaiser, H., Z. analyt. Chem. **209**, 1—18 (1965).

[30] GBl. DDR I, 1973, S. 162.

Dr. rer. nat. E. Auermann, Dr. rer. nat. J. Jacobi und Dipl.-Math. M. Kneuer, Bezirks-Hygiene-Institut Karl-Marx-Stadt, Abt. Lufthygiene, DDR-90 Karl-Marx-Stadt, Gustav-Adolf-Str. 18; Prof. Dr. Dässler, Technische Universität Dresden, Sektion Forstwirtschaft Tharandt, DDR-8223 Tharandt, Pienner Str. 8; Dipl.-Ing. K. Künzel, DDR-90 Karl-Marx-Stadt, Zeißstr. 52

Eingegangen 19. 7. 1977

Die Nahrung	22	3	1978	347—350

Zentralinstitut für Ernährung in Potsdam-Rehbrücke (Direktor: Prof. Dr. H. Haenel), Forschungszentrum für Molekularbiologie und Medizin, Akademie der Wissenschaften der DDR, und Institut für elementorganische Verbindungen der Akademie der Wissenschaften der UdSSR, Moskau (Direktor: Akademiemitglied A. N. Nesmejanov)

Zur Frage der proteolytischen Spaltung von Proteinen bei gleichzeitiger Ultrafiltration der Reaktionsprodukte

M. Friedrich, E. E. Braudo, T. W. Antonova und R. Noack

Ein proteolytischer Abbau von Casein bei gleichzeitiger Ultrafiltration der Spaltungsprodukte zeigt unter den gegebenen Bedingungen keinen höheren Spaltungsgrad als eine proteolytische Spaltung ohne Ultrafiltration oder Dialyse.
Die Ultrafiltration wurde mit DIAFLO-Membranen verschiedener Porengröße durchgeführt. Die Spaltung wurde sowohl durch E_{280} des trichloressigsäurelöslichen Überstandes als auch durch Bestimmung des Zuwachses an α-Aminostickstoff durch 2,4,6-Trinitrobenzolsulfonsäure ermittelt.

Bei der Untersuchung der enzymatischen Spaltbarkeit von Proteinen haben Bestimmungsmethoden Verbreitung gefunden, die eine Dialyse der Proteolyseprodukte beinhalten [1—4]. Damit sollte in gewisser Weise der physiologische Resorptionsprozeß simuliert werden, um eine Endprodukthemmung auf die Proteasen zu verhindern [3, 5]. Es ist noch immer unklar, in welchem Umfang die Reaktionsprodukte der endopeptidatischen Spaltung von Nahrungsproteinen die Aktivität der Proteasen tatsächlich beeinflussen.

Die Einführung unterschiedlicher Ultrafiltrationsmembranen mit definierten Porengrößen könnte zu einer genaueren Klassifizierung der für einen möglichen Hemmeffekt verantwortlichen Proteolyseendprodukte führen [6].

Methodik

Kristallisiertes Pepsin (Olajaner Chemikalienwerk, UdSSR) sowie Trypsin und Chymotrypsin (VEB Berlin-Chemie) waren Handelspräparate. Hammersten-Casein wurde nach Dunn [7] gereinigt, 2,4,6-Trinitrobenzolsulfonsäure (TNBS) nach Golumbick u. a. [8, 9] synthetisiert; Fp 195 °C. Ultrafiltrationszelle und Ultrafiltrationsmembranen UM-05, UM-2 und UM-10 waren Erzeugnisse der Fa. Amicon B. V., Niederlande.

Inkubation mit Ultrafiltration

Die Inkubation wurde in einer Ultrafiltrationszelle Modell 52 durchgeführt, die sich in einem auf 37 °C gehaltenen Wasserbad befand. In die Zelle wurden 20 ml Caseinlösung (5 mg/ml in 0,1 M Tris-HCl-Puffer pH 7,5) und 2,5 ml Enzymlösung (1 mg/ml in 10^{-3} M HCl, Trypsin: Chymotrypsin 1:1 w/w) gegeben. In Anwesenheit jeweils eines der obengenannten Filter wurde der Inkubationsansatz mit Tris-HCl-Puffer 0,1 M pH 7,5 gespült (0,8 ml/min), bis das Filtrat das vierfache Volumen des Inkubationsansatzes erreichte (80 ml in ca. 100 min). Das Volumen innerhalb der Ultrafiltrationszelle blieb mit 20 ml unverändert. In Vorversuchen wurde nachgewiesen, daß nach 100 min die Proteolyse nahezu vollständig abgeschlossen ist. Eine Erhöhung der Enzym-Substrat-Relation von 1:40 (in vorliegendem Inkubationsansatz) auf 1:10 erbrachte keinen höheren Proteolysegrad. Nach Beendigung des Versuches wurden aliquote Teile von Ultrafiltrationsrückstand bzw. von Filtrat (1 Vol. Rückstand bzw. 4 Vol. Filtrat) sowohl getrennt als auch im Gemisch mit Trichloressigsäure (TCE) versetzt (5% Endkonzentration). Inkubationsansätzen ohne Ultrafiltration wurden gleichfalls entsprechende Proben entnommen und mit TCE versetzt. Nach sämtlichen Inkubationsansätzen war der TCE-fällbare Anteil sehr gering, er betrug ca. 1–2% der eingesetzten Proteinmenge. Der TCE-lösliche Anteil repräsentiert danach die Gesamtheit des eingesetzten Proteins.

Inkubation mit Dialyse

Die Untersuchungen zur Proteolyse unter den Bedingungen der nacheinanderfolgenden Einwirkung von 1. Pepsin und 2. einem Trypsin-Chymotrypsin-Gemisch (1:1 w/w) wurden nach der Methode von SLONIMSKIJ u. a. [10] durchgeführt. Im Gegensatz zur Ultrafiltration wird der Boden des Inkubationsgefäßes mit einer Zellglasmembran von dem äußeren Flüssigkeitsraum abgetrennt. Der Übertritt der Proteolysespaltprodukte in das Dialysat erfolgt hierbei nur durch einfache Diffusion. Die Volumenverhältnisse zwischen Inkubationslösung und Dialyseflüssigkeit während der Pepsinverdauung betragen 1:4 und während der anschließenden Trypsin/Chymotrypsin-Verdauung 1:2,3. Zur Analyse werden, wie oben angegeben, aliquote Teile des Inkubationsansatzes mit TCE behandelt und der TCE-lösliche Anteil untersucht.

Analytik

Die Bestimmung der TCE-löslichen Anteile wurde nach 2 Methoden durchgeführt:

1. Extinktionsmessung bei 280 nm nach KUNITZ [11],
2. Reaktion mit TNBS zur Bestimmung des α-Aminostickstoffs [12, 13].

Die letztere Methode wurde in 2 Varianten erprobt:

1. Messung der Extinktion nach beendeter Reaktion im sauren pH-Bereich bei 340 nm [12],
2. Messung der Extinktion nach beendeter Reaktion im alkalischen pH-Bereich unter Zusatz von Methanol bei 420 nm [14].

Zur Bestimmung wird 0,1 ml Probe (TCE-Überstand, 5% TCE) mit 1,0 ml TNBS-Lösung (0,2 g TNBS/ml 0,2 M Boraxlösung pH 9,15) versetzt (= 1,1 ml von pH 8,55). Man inkubiert die Lösung 30 min bei 37 °C, gibt 0,5 ml 1 N HCl (Variante 1; End-pH = 1,1) bzw. 2,0 ml Methanol (Variante 2) zu und mißt am VSU 1 in 1 cm-Küvetten.

Anhand von Aminosäuren (Gly, Leu, Glu, Lys, Thr, Phe) und Peptiden (Gly-phe, Gly-gly-gly, Leu-gly-gly und red. Glutathion) wurden beide Varianten verglichen. Es zeigte sich, daß der saure pH-Wert einen farbstabilisierenden Einfluß besitzt. Die relativen Farbausbeuten der verwendeten Aminosäuren und Peptide sind nach beiden Varianten ähnlich und betragen im Vergleich zu Leucin nach

Variante 1: $100 \pm 22\%$
Variante 2: $119 \pm 33\%$.

Resultate und Diskussion

Tab. 1 zeigt den Proteolysegrad im Ultrafiltrationsexperiment als Relation zwischen der Spaltung mit und ohne Ultrafiltration. Der Anteil der Proteolyseprodukte wurde sowohl im Gemisch aliquoter Teile von Inkubationsflüssigkeit und Ultrafiltrat als auch als Summe der Einzelbestimmungen beider Kompartments ermittelt. Die Resultate waren übereinstimmend.

Tab. 1 zeigt weiterhin, daß mit der Erhöhung der Membrandurchlässigkeit die Menge und die Größe der Peptide erwartungsgemäß im Filtrat ansteigt. Der Anstieg der Menge ist aus dem Zuwachs an α-Aminostickstoff zu erkennen (21% auf 44%) und

Tabelle 1
Proteolyse von Casein durch ein Trypsin/Chymotrypsin-Gemisch bei gleichzeitiger Ultrafiltration der Spaltprodukte

Membran	Anzahl der Versuche	Relation $\frac{\text{Inkubation mit Ultrafiltration}}{\text{Inkubation ohne Ultrafiltration}}$		Prozentualer Anteil der in das Ultrafiltrat übergetretenen Spaltprodukte	
		Analyse durch ΔE_{280}	Analyse mit TNBS	Analyse durch ΔE_{280}	Analyse mit TNBS
UM-05	2	1,03	1,03	21	21
UM-2	3	0,96±0,10	1,03±0,11	38±11	33±10
UM-10	3	0,97±0,04	1,04±0,08	54± 1	44± 3

die Zunahme der Peptidgröße aus dem Anstieg der Relation Analysenwert ΔE_{280} zu Analysenwert TNBS (1 auf 1,23). Trotz filtrierbarer Spaltproduktanteile von 21% (Membran UM-05) bis zu 54% (Membran UM-10) sind keine Unterschiede des Proteolysegrades bezüglich einer Inkubation ohne Eliminierung der Spaltprodukte festzustellen.

Der absolute Spaltungsgrad des Caseins nach diesen Inkubationen betrug ca. 17%, wenn der α-Aminostickstoffgehalt des Caseins nach salzsaurer Totalhydrolyse als 100% angenommen wird.

Keine Unterschiede zwischen einer Inkubation ohne Dialyse bzw. Dialyse unter Anwendung von Zellglas als Dialysemembran zeigt Tab. 2. Hierbei ist zu sehen, daß die Spaltung durch Pepsin und durch die Pankreasproteasen Trypsin-Chymotrypsin bei gleichzeitiger Dialyse nicht gefördert wird. Wie im Ultrafiltrationsexperiment liegt der Grenzwert der Spaltung wiederum bei ca. 17%.

Tabelle 2
Proteolyse von Casein durch aufeinanderfolgende Einwirkung von Pepsin und Trypsin/Chymotrypsin-Gemisch mit und ohne Dialyse durch Zellglasmembran

Proteolyse-bedingungen	Anzahl der Versuche	Prozentualer Proteolysegrad nach Inkubation mit	
		Pepsin	Trypsin/ Chymotrypsin
ohne Dialyse	4	4,8±0,2	17,7±0,6
mit Dialyse	4	5,5±0,1	16,6±0,05

Diese Versuche machen deutlich, daß bei Substratkonzentrationen bis mindestens 5 mg/ml im Inkubationsansatz und Spaltungsraten bis mindestens 17% eine Endprodukthemmung auf die Endopeptidasen Trypsin bzw. Chymotrypsin nicht eintritt und eine Dialyse für derartige Modellversuche zur Verdaulichkeit nicht notwendig ist.

Summary

M. FRIEDRICH, E. E. BRAUDO, T. W. ANTONOVA and R. NOACK: On the question of combining the proteolysis of proteins with the ultrafiltration of the reaction products

Under the experimental conditions chosen, the degree of cleavage achieved by combining the proteolysis of casein with the ultrafiltration of the decomposition products was not greater than that obtained from the proteolytic degradation without ultrafiltration or dialysis.

Ultrafiltration was performed by means of DIAFLO membranes of varying pore sizes. The cleavage was evidenced by determining both the E_{280} value of the TCA-soluble supernatant and the increase in α-amino nitrogen (reaction with 2.4.6-trinitrobenzenesulphonic acid).

Резюме

М. Фридрих, Е. Е. Браудо, Т. В. Антонова и Р. Ноакк: К вопросу протеолитического расщепления белков при одновременной ультрафильтрации продуктов реакции

При протеолитическом расщеплении казеина и одновременной ультрафильтрации продуктов распада в данных условиях не удается обнаружить более высокую степень расщенления чем при протеолитическом расщеплении без ультрафильтрации или диализа.

Ультрафильтрация проводилась с помощью DIAFLO-мембран с различной величиной пор. О расщеплении судили как с помощью E_{280} растворимого в трихлоруксусной кислоте надсадке, так и путем определения увеличения α-аминоазота с помощью 2,4,6-тринитробензолсулфоновой кислоты.

Literatur

[1] BALDWIN, R. R., J. R. LOWRY u. R. THIESSEN, jr., Food Res. **16**, 107 (1951).
[2] MAURON, J., F. MOTTU, E. BUJARD u. R. H. EGLI, Arch. Biochem. Biophysics **59**, 433 (1955).
[3] PRAHL, L., u. K. TÄUFEL, Nahrung **10**, 31 (1966).
[4] POKROVSKIJ, A. A., u. I. D. JERTANOV, Voprosy Pitanija **24**, 38 (1965).
[5] TSCHERNIKOW, M. P., Biochimija **28**, 285 (1963).
[6] Firmenschrift: Ultrafiltration with Diaflo-Membranes for Laboratory and Clinical Uses. Catalog and Applications Guide, Amicon N. V. Oosterhout (N. B.) Holland, 1972.
[7] DUNN, H. S., u. K. E. CARTER, Biochemical Preparations, Vol. 1, p. 22, John Wiley and Sons Inc., New York.1949.
[8] GOLUMBICK, S., J. S. FRUTON u. M. BERGMANN, J. org. Chem. **11**, 534 (1946).
[9] HEILKAMP, G. K., u. D. J. PETTITT, Org. Synthesis **46**, 124 (1966).
[10] SLONIMSKIJ, G. L., E. E. BRAUDO, I. D. JERTANOW, W. B. TOLSTOGUSOV, E. S. BONDAREVA u. I. G. PLAŠČINA, Voprosy Pitanija **29**, 25 (1970).
[11] KUNITZ, M., J. gen. Physiol. **30**, 29 (1947).
[12] LANGNER, J., S. ANSORGE, P. BOHLEY, H. KIRSCHKE u. H. HANSON, Acta biol. med. german. **26**, 935 (1971).
[13] SATAKE, K., T. OKUYAMA, M. OHASHI u. T. SHINODA, J. Biochem. [Tokyo] **47**, 654 (1960).
[14] MOKRASH, L. C., Analyt. Biochem. **18**, 64 (1967).

Dr. M. FRIEDRICH und Prof. Dr. R. NOACK, Zentralinstitut für Ernährung, 1505 Bergholz-Rehbrücke, Arthur-Scheunert-Allee 114—116, und Dr. E. E. BRAUDO und T. W. ANTONOVA, Institut für elementorganische Verbindungen der Akademie der Wissenschaften der UdSSR, 117813 Moskau W-312, ul. Wawilowa 28

Eingegangen 5. 9. 1977

Die Nahrung	22	3	1978	351—355

Bereich Lebensmittelchemie der Sektion Chemie der Humboldt-Universität zu Berlin
(Leiter: Prof. Dr. Cl. FRANZKE), DDR

Studien zur Glyceridstruktur von Fetten[1]
11. Mitt. Strukturuntersuchungen an ausgewählten Nußfetten mit Hilfe von Lipasen

Cl. FRANZKE, J. KROLL und R. GÖBEL

Mit Hilfe der Pankreaslipase und der Lipase von *Geotrichum candidum* werden Fettsäureverteilung und Glyceridklassenzusammensetzung von Erdnuß-, Walnuß-, Haselnuß- Paranuß- und Cashewnußfett bestimmt. Sowohl Fettsäureverteilung als auch Glyceridklassenzusammensetzung sind mit denen anderer Pflanzenfette, die eine entsprechende Gesamtfettsäurezusammensetzung besitzen, vergleichbar.

Während die Fettsäurezusammensetzung der meisten Nußfette bekannt ist, gibt es über Fettsäureverteilung sowie Zusammensetzung der Glyceridklassen nur wenige Hinweise in der Literatur [1—9]. Lediglich für Erdnuß- und Haselnußfett liegen entsprechende Angaben vor [10, 11].

Ziel dieser Arbeit ist es, die Fettsäureverteilung und Glyceridklassenzusammensetzung von 5 ausgewählten Nußfetten, nämlich von Erdnuß (*Arachis hypogaea L.*), Haselnuß (*Corylus avellana L.*), Walnuß (*Juglaus regia L.*), Paranuß (*Bertholletia excelsa H. B. K.*) und Cashewnuß (*Anacardium occidentale L.*) mit Hilfe von enzymatischen Methoden zu bestimmen.

Versuchssubstanzen und Methoden

Die wesentlichen Kennzahlen für die durch Extraktion mit Diäthyläther aus den zerkleinerten Samen gewonnenen Nußfette sind in Tab. 1 zusammengefaßt dargestellt.

Tabelle 1
Kennzahlen der eingesetzten Nußfette

Fett	Verseifungszahl	Säurezahl	Peroxidzahl [mÄqu/kg]	Unverseifbares [%]
Erdnuß	189,0	0,2	0,6	0,9
Haselnuß	193,1	0,3	0,4	0,5
Walnuß	190,6	0,5	1,0	0,4
Paranuß	191,9	0,2	0,4	0,8
Cashewnuß	190,7	0,2	0,6	0,5

Die Lipolyse der Fettsubstrate mit Pankreaslipase und mit der Lipase von *Geotrichum candidum*, die dünnschichtchromatographische Auftrennung der Lipolyseprodukte sowie die gaschromatographische Analyse der Methylester werden nach den bereits von uns beschriebenen Verfahren durchgeführt [13].

[1] 10. Mitt. Nahrung **21**, 367—368 (1977).

Die Berechnung der Hauptglyceridklassen aus den ermittelten Daten nach Hydrolyse mit Pankreaslipase erfolgt auf der Grundlage der Hypothese der 1,3-random-2-random-distribution nach VAN DER WAL [12]. Die direkte Bestimmung der Glyceridzusammensetzung mit Hilfe der Lipase von *Geotrichum candidum* wird nach der bereits mitgeteilten Methode durchgeführt [13].

Ergebnisse und Diskussion

In Tab. 2 sind die Fettsäurezusammensetzung der Nußfette sowie die Fettsäurezusammensetzung der nach Hydrolyse mit Pankreaslipase erhaltenen und dünnschichtchromatographisch isolierten 2-Monoglyceride zusammengefaßt dargestellt.

Aus Tab. 2 ist eine Anreicherung der Summe der ungesättigten Fettsäuren in der 2-Position der Triglyceride, die typisch ist für pflanzliche Samenfette, ersichtlich; lediglich bei Cashewnußfett ist diese Anreicherung nicht mehr als eindeutig zu bezeichnen. Die von BROCKERHOFF u. a. [10] bzw. BAZAN u. a. [11] für Erdnuß- bzw. Haselnußfett bestimmte Fettsäureverteilung kann bestätigt werden.

Die auf der Grundlage der in Tab. 2 aufgezeigten Ergebnisse berechnete Glyceridklassenzusammensetzung der Nußfette ist in Tab. 3 dargestellt.

Tabelle 2
Fettsäurezusammensetzung der Gesamttriglyceride sowie der 2-Monoglyceride nach Pankreaslipasehydrolyse

Fett	Fraktion	Fettsäurezusammensetzung						
		$C_{14:0}$	$C_{16:0}$	$C_{18:0}$	$C_{18:1}$	$C_{18:2}$	$C_{18:3}$ + $C_{20:1}$	$C_{22:0}$
Erdnuß	Gesamt-TG	0,8	11,2	2,3	40,8	40,9	3,0	1,0
	2-Monoglyceride	0,4	5,1	1,6	32,2	60,0	0,5	0,2
Haselnuß	Gesamt-TG		5,3	2,0	80,8	11,9		
	2-Monoglyceride		1,9	0,9	79,7	17,5		
Walnuß	Gesamt-TG		11,1	1,8	22,1	43,8	21,2	
	2-Monoglyceride		4,9	0,8	20,0	62,0	12,3	
Paranuß	Gesamt-TG		14,6	9,1	29,3	47,0		
	2-Monoglyceride		3,6	3,4	38,4	54,6		
Cashewnuß	Gesamt-TG		10,3	7,3	61,1	21,3		
	2-Monoglyceride		8,3	5,1	58,9	27,7		

TG = Triglyceride

Tabelle 3
Glyceridklassenzusammensetzung der Nußfette, berechnet nach der 1,3-random-2-random distribution

Nußart	Glyceridklassenzusammensetzung [Mol%]					
	GGG*	UGG**	GUG	GUU	UGU	UUU
Erdnuß	0,3	2,3	3,4	28,6	4,8	60,6
Haselnuß	Sp.	0,5	0,9	16,8	2,3	79,5
Walnuß	0,2	1,6	2,5	25,9	4,0	65,8
Paranuß	0,7	3,0	9,6	40,7	3,2	42,8
Cashewnuß	0,5	4,2	3,3	27,4	8,6	56,0

*G = gesättigte Fettsäuren
**U = ungesättigte Fettsäuren

Entsprechend der Fettsäurezusammensetzung der Nußfette ist der Anteil der triungesättigten Glyceride (UUU) und der unsymmetrischen monogesättigten-diungesättigten Glyceride (GUU) mit insgesamt 83—95% (Tab. 3) außerordentlich hoch.

Zur direkten Bestimmung der Glyceridklassenzusammensetzung werden die Nußfette mit Lipase von *Geotrichum candidum*, einem fettsäurespezifisch wirkenden Enzym (spaltet bevorzugt cis-9-ungesättigte Fettsäuren aus Glyceridsubstraten ab), inkubiert. Die Fettsäurezusammensetzung der dünnschichtchromatographisch aufgetrennten Lipolyseprodukte ist in Tab. 4 wiedergegeben.

Aus den in Tab. 4 dargestellten Ergebnissen wird nach der von uns veröffentlichten Methode [13] direkt die Glyceridzusammensetzung berechnet (Tab. 5).

Unter Berücksichtigung der Tatsache, daß die Lipase von *Geotrichum candidum* eine absolute Spezifität für cis-9-ungesättigte Fettsäuren nicht besitzt und daß bei der zweifachen Dünnschichtchromatographie der Lipolyseprodukte Veränderungen der Fettsäurezusammensetzung durch Autoxydation nicht ausgeschlossen werden können, sind die in Tab. 5 aufgeführten Ergebnisse annähernd mit den auf der Grundlage der Pankreaslipasehydrolyse berechneten Daten (Tab. 3) vergleichbar. Unterschiede bestehen im wesentlichen in dem jeweils um ca. 7—12% geringeren Gehalt an triungesättigten Glyceriden (UUU) und in dem höheren Gehalt an isomeren monoungesättigten-digesättigten Glyceriden (UGG, GUG).

Tabelle 4
Fettsäurezusammensetzung der unter Einwirkung der Lipase von *Geotrichum candidum* gebildeten Reaktionsprodukte

Fett	Fraktion	Fettsäurezusammensetzung (Mol%)						
		$C_{14:0}$	$C_{16:0}$	$C_{18:0}$	$C_{18:1}$	$C_{18:2}$	$C_{18:3}$ + $C_{20:1}$	$C_{22:0}$
Erdnuß	1,3-DG	0,6	20,0	5,0	36,3	24,8	9,4	3,9
	1,2-DG	0,4	12,0	4,0	34,0	45,0	2,6	2,0
	1-MG	1,4	26,2	10,7	29,0	15,8	11,7	5,2
	2-MG	0,6	5,1	1,6	36,2	45,4	10,5	0,6
Haselnuß	1,3-DG		10,3	4,2	76,1	9,4		
	1,2-DG		6,4	2,2	80,5	10,9		
	1-MG		15,1	5,3	69,7	9,9		
	2-MG		2,5	1,7	83,8	12,0		
Walnuß	1,3-DG		16,3	4,3	14,1	52,3	13,0	
	1,2-DG		13,4	2,0	14,2	57,5	12,9	
	1-MG		29,7	10,4	20,4	36,3	3,2	
	2-MG		5,1	2,8	25,1	57,0	10,0	
Paranuß	1,3-DG		27,9	17,4	28,2	26,5		
	1,2-DG		16,0	8,8	30,8	44,4		
	1-MG		33,3	30,4	16,8	19,5		
	2-MG		6,5	4,3	34,2	55,0		
Cashewnuß	1,3-DG		19,0	16,2	44,1	20,7		
	1,2-DG		12,2	8,0	54,5	25,3		
	1-MG		22,7	19,0	39,9	18,4		
	2-MG		8,7	4,2	65,7	21,4		

MG = Monoglyceride
DG = Diglyceride

Tabelle 5
Glyceridklassenzusammensetzung der Nußfette, bestimmt aus den Daten der Hydrolyse mit Lipase von *Geotrichum candidum*

Nußart	Glyceridklassenzusammensetzung [Mol%]					
	GGG*	UGG	GUG	GUU	IGU	UUU
Erdnuß	—	4,4	7,9	30,0	5,5	52,2
Haselnuß	—	4,3	9,6	15,6	3,2	67,3
Walnuß	—	4,4	0,8	30,7	6,1	58,0
Paranuß	—	7,8	15,1	35,7	6,1	35,3
Cashewnuß	—	2,6	8,5	29,1	9,0	50,8

* nicht bestimmbar mit dieser Methode

Insgesamt gesehen, sind die untersuchten Nußfette in bezug auf Fettsäureverteilung und Glyceridklassenzusammensetzung mit anderen Pflanzenfetten, die eine entsprechende Gesamtfettsäurezusammensetzung besitzen, vergleichbar.

Summary

Cl. FRANZKE, J. KROLL and R. GÖBEL: Studies on the glyceride structure of fats. Part XI. Structure analyses of selected nut fats, using lipases

Using pancreatic lipase and the lipase of *Geotrichum candidum*, the authors determined the fatty acid pattern and the glyceride structure of peanut, filbert, walnut, Brazil nut and cashew-nut fats. Bot the fatty acid pattern and the glyceride structure were comparable to those of other vegetable fats of corresponding total fatty acid composition.

Резоме

Кл. Францке, Й. Кролль и Р. Гебель: Изучение глицеридной структуры жиров. Сообщ. 11. Исследование структуры избранных ореховых масел с помощью липаз

С помощью панкреатической липазы и липазы *Geotrichum candidum* определялись распределение жирных кислот и состав глицеридных классов в маслах арахиса, фундука, грецкого ореха, американского ореха и орехов кешью. Наблюдается сходство как по распределению жирных кислот так и по составу глицеридных кдассов с другими растительными маслами, обладающими соответственным составом общих жирных кислот.

Literatur

[1] ZÜRCHER, K., und H. HADORN, Mitt. Gebiete Lebensmittelunters. Hyg. **66**, 191 (1975).
[2] BULNINSKI, R., Bromat. Chem. Toksykol. **7**, 405 (1974).
[3] SUBBARAN, M. R., und C. G. YOUNGS, J. Amer. Oil Chemist's Soc. **44**, 425 (1967).
[4] MEHRAN, M., J. Amer. Oil Chemist's Soc. **51**, 477 (1974).
[5] KAUFMANN, H. P., und J. BAROC, Fette, Seifen, Anstrichmittel **69**, 437 (1967).
[6] SIETZ, F. G., Fette, Seifen, Anstrichmittel **71**, 446 (1969).
[7] SEIDEMANN, J., Seifen, Öle, Fette, Wachse **99**, 302 (1973).
[8] BANCHER, E., J. WASHÜTTL und H. J. GOLLER, Seifen, Öle, Fette, Wachse **98**, 555 (1972).
[9] BARTHEL, G., G. LASKAWY und W. GROSCH, Dtsch. Lebensm. Rdsch. **70**, 201 (1974).
[10] BROCKERHOFF, H., und M. YURKOWSKI, J. Lipid Res. **7**. 62 (1966).
[11] BAZAN, E., C. PETRONICI, M. PAUSSO und V. AVERNA, Riv. ital. Sostanze grasse **52**, 230 (1975).
[12] Van der WAL, R. J., J. Amer. Oil Chemist's Soc. **37**, 18 (1960).
[13] KROLL, J., und Cl. FRANZKE, Fette, Seifen, Anstrichmittel **76**, 385 (1974).

Prof. Dr. Cl. FRANZKE, Bereich Lebensmittelchemie der Sektion Chemie der Humboldt-Universität zu Berlin, DDR — 112 Berlin, Goethestr. 54

Eingegangen 21. 9. 1977

Die Nahrung	22	3	1978	355—358

Zentralstelle für Futtermittelprüfung und Fütterung Halle-Lettin
(Direktor: Dr. KNAPE), DDR

Flammenphotometrische Natrium- und Calcium-schnellbestimmung in Futtermitteln (Wissenschaftlicher Kurzbericht)

J. v. LENGERKEN und M. ZEIDLER

Die Produktivität bei der flammenphotometrischen Na- und Ca-Bestimmung wird wesentlich durch die Art der Probenaufbereitung beeinflußt. Anliegen und Ziel unserer Untersuchungen war es aus diesem Grunde, die Eignung des spektrochemischen Puffers nach EBERT [1] für die flammenphotometrische Na- und Ca-Bestimmung in Futtermitteln zu prüfen und die sich ergebenden einfach durchzuführenden flammenphotometrischen Bestimmungen mit einer von uns erarbeiteten Schnellmineralisierung [2] zu kombinieren.

Untersuchungen zur Methode

Alle Bestimmungen erfolgten mit einem Flapho 4 vom VEB Carl Zeiß Jena (bei den Versuchen zur Ermittlung der Einflußgrößen wurde nach der Ausschlagmethode gemessen). Untersucht werden sollte der Einfluß des Mineralisierungsgemisches (M) und der Mineralstoffe. Letzterer wurde global durch Zugabe von 1—3 ml einer synthetischen Aschelösung (MSL) zum Mineralisat, die in der Zusammensetzung und Menge einem 1—3fachen durchschnittlichen Aschegehalt des Futtermittels ohne Na- bzw. Ca-Zusatz entsprach, geprüft.

Aus Abb. 1 und 2 ist zu ersehen, daß Schwefelsäure und Mineralstoffe in unterschiedlichem Maße auf die Lage der Eichkurven Einfluß nehmen. Diese Einflüsse werden, wie aus den gleichen Abbildungen zu entnehmen ist, durch die Zugabe von Pufferlösung (P) und des Mineralisierungsgemisches (M) zur Probe und zum sog. Blindansatz kompensiert.

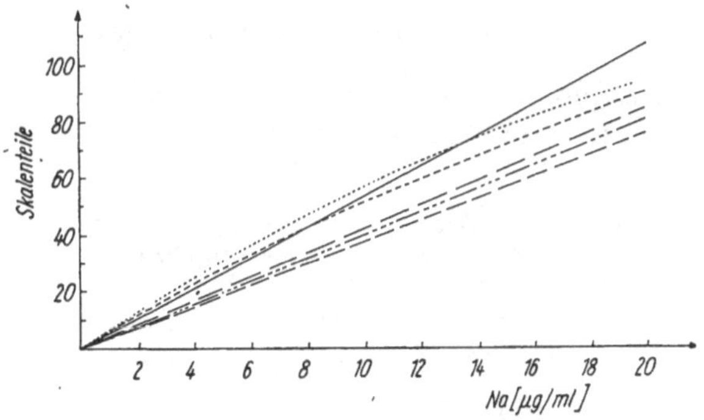

Abb. 1. Einfluß des Mineralisierungsgemisches (M) und der synthetischen Aschelösung (MSL) auf die flammenphotometrische Natriumbestimmung

——— Na-Standardlösung, — — Na-Standardlösung + M, — · — · Na-Standardlösung + M + 1 ml MSL, - - - - Na-Standardlösung + M + 2 ml MSL, ······ Na-Standardlösung + M + 3 ml MSL, — - - - — Na-Standardlösung + M + 1-3 ml MSL + P

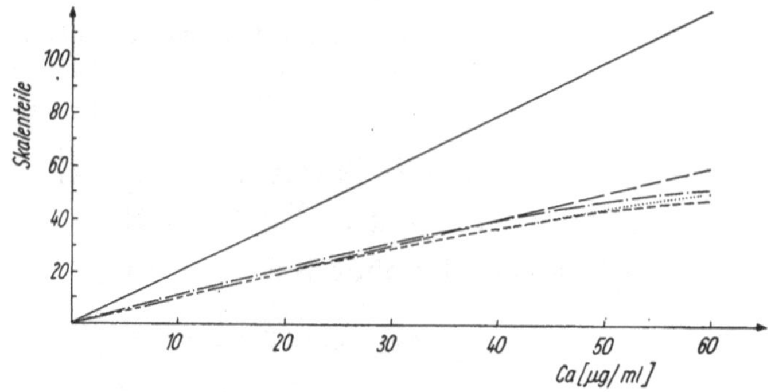

Abb. 2. Einfluß des Mineralisierungsgemisches (M) und der synthetischen Aschelösung (MSL) auf die flammenphotometrische Calciumbestimmung

——— Ca-Standardlösung, — — Ca-Standardlösung + M; Ca-Standardlösung + M + 1-3 MSL + P, —·—· Ca-Standardlösung + M + 1 ml MSL, ---- Ca-Standardlösung + M + 2 ml MSL, ······ Ca Standardlösung + M + 3 ml MSL

Vorschrift zur Natriumbestimmung

300 mg (500 mg) der Proben werden in 50 ml (100 ml) Meßkolben nacheinander mit 2 ml (4 ml) H_2O_2, 30%ig, und 3 ml (4 ml) H_2SO_4, konz., versetzt. (Vorsicht! Arbeitsschutzanordnung beachten!). Die Mineralisierung der Probe ist nach Selbsterwärmung in ca. 1 min beendet. Nach Abkühlen wird mit dest. Wasser zur Eichmarke aufgefüllt und umgeschüttelt. Hierauf wird ein aliquoter Teil von 1 ml mit 4 ml verdünnter Pufferlösung (Pufferlösung und dest. Wasser im Verhältnis 1 : 4) verdünnt und am Flammenphotometer gegen einen Blindansatz, der die verwendeten Chemikalien enthält (Mineralisierungsgemisch und Pufferlösung), gemessen.

Die Standardkurven in den Bereichen von 0—20 µg Na/ml bzw. 0—250 µg Ca/ml werden wie bei den Proben unter Zusatz von Schwefelsäure und verdünnter Pufferlösung aufgestellt.

Zusammensetzung der Pufferlösung

0,767 g KH_2PO_4 in 30 ml 20%iger HCl, 0,474 g $AlCl_3 \cdot 6\,H_2O$, 101,36 g $MgSO_4 \cdot 7\,H_2O$ und 1 ml Brij, 30%ig, oder eine äquivalente Menge einer waschaktiven Substanz, z. B. Cetyltrimethylammoniumbromid, in 1 l H_2O. Durch die Zugabe von waschaktiven Substanzen zur Meßlösung lassen sich die Zerstäuberleistung und Reproduzierbarkeit der Messung entscheidend verbessern.

Überprüfungsergebnisse

Die Richtigkeit der Ergebnisse dieser Vorschrift wurde durch sog. Wiederfindungsversuche geprüft, deren Resultate aus Tab. 1 und 2 zu ersehen sind. In Tab. 3 erfolgt

Tabelle 1
Ergebnisse von Na-Wiederfindungsversuchen bei Mischfutter und Natronlaugestrohpelletproben

Na-Gehalt der Proben $\bar{x}$ [g/kg]	Na-Gehalt nach Zusatz von 2,5 g Na/kg [g/kg]	Wiederfindung [%]	Na-Gehalt nach Zusatz von 5 g Na/kg [g/kg]	Wiederfindung [%]	Na-Gehalt nach Zusatz von 10 g Na/kg [g/kg]	Wiederfindung [%]
3,16	5,50	102	8,13	100	13,42	98
9,43	12,13	98	14,30	101	19,65	99
18,75	21,30	99	23,23	102	28,50	101
22,55	24,80	101	27,80	99	32,06	102
31,12	33,62	100	36,56	98	—	—

Tabelle 2
Ergebnisse von Ca-Wiederfindungsversuchen bei Mischfuttermitteln

Ca-Gehalt der Proben $\bar{x}$ [g/kg]	Ca-Gehalt nach Zusatz von 5 g Ca/kg [g/kg]	Wiederfindung [%]	Ca-Gehalt nach Zusatz von 10 g Ca/kg [g/kg]	Wiederfindung [%]
2,20	7,06	97	12,06	99
5,80	10,80	100	15,86	101
7,61	12,74	103	17,75	101
8,42	13,48	101	18,42	100
16,63	21,56	99	26,69	101

Tabelle 3
Ergebnisse von Ca-Bestimmungen nach der vorgeschlagenen flammenphotometrischen Methode im Vergleich zur TGL 80-21875/10 bei Mischfuttermitteln

Futtermittel	Ca-Gehalt [g/kg] ermittelt nach der	
	flammenphotometrischen Methode	TGL-Methode
Ferkelaufzuchtfutter	7,8	7,7
	5,8	6,2
Sauenfutter	9,8	9,9
	8,8	9,4
Broilermastalleinfutter	10,8	11,2
	11,8	11,9
	10,6	10,1
	10,8	11,5
Legehennenalleinfutter	17,6	17,3
	29,3	30,0
	33,4	33,8
	33,6	33,2

Tabelle 4
Ergebnisse zur Reproduzierbarkeit der Natriumbestimmung bei Mischfutter und Natronlaugestrohpelletproben (n = 10)

Probe	$\bar{X}$	S_1	V_1	S_2	V_2
1	3,16	0,104	3,3	0,09	2,8
2	9,43	0,251	2,7	0,12	1,3
3	18,75	0,516	2,8	0,25	1,3
4	24,78	0,605	2,4	0,29	1,2
5	31,12	0,690	2,0	0,30	1,0

$$S = \pm \sqrt{\frac{(\bar{x}_i - x)^2}{n - 1}}$$

S_1; V_1 = für Parallelbest. aus verschiedenen Mineralisaten

$$V = \frac{S \cdot 100}{x}$$

S_2; V_2 = für Parallelbest. aus jeweils einem Mineralisat

$\bar{X}$ = durchschnittlicher Na- bzw. Ca-Gehalt [g/kg]
S = Streuung
V = Variationskoeffizient

ein Vergleich zur Calciumbestimmung nach der komplexometrischen Methode nach TGL 80-21875/10. In Verbindung mit den Ergebnissen der Versuche zur Ermittlung der Reproduzierbarkeit, dargestellt in Tab. 4 und 5, zeigen sie die Anwendbarkeit dieser Bestimmungsmethoden für die uns im Zusammenhang mit dem Natronlauge- bzw. Natriumchlorideinsatz interessierenden Futtermittel. Der Vorteil der Methoden liegt in dem geringen Zeitaufwand je Bestimmung und in einer hohen Arbeitsproduktivität.

Tabelle 5
Ergebnisse zur Reproduzierbarkeit der Ca-Bestimmung bei Mischfuttermitteln (n = 10)

Probe	$\bar{X}$	S_1	V_1	S_2	V_2
1	2,20	0,10	4,5	0,06	2,7
2	5,80	0,12	2,1	0,07	1,2
3	7,61	0,15	2,0	0,07	0,9
4	8,42	0,17	2,0	0,09	1,1
5	16,63	0,32	1,9	0,10	0,9

Literatur

[1] EBERT, K., Z. Landw. Vers.-Unters.-Wesen **10**, 329 (1964).
[2] LENGERKEN, J. v., V. MÜLLER und H. WETTERAU, Nahrung **18**, 551 (1974).

Dr. rer. nat. J. v. LENGERKEN und Prüfing. MARTINA ZEIDLER, Zentralstelle für Futtermittelprüfung und Fütterung, DDR-4025 Halle-Lettin, Schiepziger Str. 35

Eingegangen 17. 10. 1977

Die Nahrung	22	3	1978	359–373

Kurznachrichten

BÜCHER UND ZEITSCHRIFTEN

G. THIESSEN und H. THIESSEN: MICROSPECTROPHOTOMETRIC CELL ANALYSIS. Progress in Histochemistry and Cytochemistry Vol. 9, No. 4. 158 Seiten, 92 Abb. und 14 Tab. Gustav Fischer Verlag, Stuttgart–New York 1977. Preis: 74,– DM.

Die Autoren haben sich methodisch und theoretisch mit der mikrospektrophotometrischen Zellanalyse jahrelang befaßt und durch die Entwicklung eines digitalen Mikrospektrophotometers mit transformierter Darstellung der Meßergebnisse (CYTOS-System) große Verdienste auf diesem Gebiet erworben. Das Buch stellt eine Art Resumé dar. Es enthält eine detaillierte Beschreibung des Aufbaus und der Funktion des CYTOS-Systems. Für eine spätere praktische Anwendung bietet es die Möglichkeit, Diagnosen zu stellen, wo nur wenig Zellmaterial zur Verfügung steht und wo vor allem gezielt die individuelle intrazelluläre Substanzverteilung, die Kinetik und der Metabolismus für die Klassifikation von zytologischen Objekten von Interesse ist. Als Beispiel werden Ergebnisse an Spermatozoen als Referenzobjekte und Untersuchungen an Gewebezellkulturen nach UV-Bestrahlung mit gezielter Analyse der Chromosomenaberrationen methodenkritisch diskutiert. D. W. R. BLEYL

J. LEHMANN: CHEMIE DER KOHLENHYDRATE, MONOSACCHARIDE UND DERIVATE. VII und 279 Seiten, 332 Schemata, 12 Tab., Georg Thieme Verlag, Stuttgart 1976. Preis: 24,80 DM.

Das vorliegende Buch erscheint im Rahmen der Reihe „Thieme Taschenlehrbuch der organischen Chemie, B. Spezielle Gebiete". Dementsprechend ist es nach Gliederung und Inhalt als Lehrbuch angelegt und umfaßt folgende Aspekte aus der Chemie der Monosaccharide und ihrer Derivate: Struktur der Monosaccharide, Eigenschaften und Verhalten der Monosaccharide als Carbonylverbindungen oder cyklische Acetale sowie als Polyole, strukturelle Veränderungen durch starke Mineralsäuren und Basen und schließlich ausgewählte Untersuchungsmethoden sowie einen Exkurs in die systematische Nomenklatur. Bei strenger Orientierung auf den neueren Erkenntnisstand und unter besonderer Berücksichtigung stereochemischer Aspekte wird in verständlicher Darstellung und prägnanter Kürze ein umfangreicher Wissensstoff vermittelt. Durch die Kürze in der Behandlung von Stoffklassen und deren spezifische Eigenschaften bedingt, werden die übergeordneten Prinzipien der chemischen Umsetzungen in einer dem Verständnis der Monosaccharidreaktionen förderlichen Weise hervorgehoben. Weiterhin wünschenswert wären eine theoretische Behandlung der enzymatisch gesteuerten Monosaccharidreaktionen sowie eine stärkere Berücksichtigung der enzymatischen Untersuchungsmethoden. F. SCHIERBAUM

SPEZIFITÄT UND KONTROLLREAKTIONEN IN DER HISTOCHEMIE. Herausgegeben von Ch. PILGRIM. 282 Seiten, 125 Abb. und 39 Tab. Acta histochem. Suppl-Bd. XVIII. VEB Gustav Fischer Verlag, Jena 1977. Preis: DDR 77,– M; Ausland 97,– M.

Der Suppl.Bd. gibt die Verhandlungen der Gesellschaft für Histochemie auf ihrem XVIII. Symposium vom 8.–11. Oktober 1975 wieder. Das Symposium war in 3 Workshops unterteilt: 1. Spezifität und Kontrollreaktionen in der Kohlenhydrathistochemie, 2. Spezifität histochemischer Enzymnachweise und Kontrollreaktionen und 3. Zytochemische Merkmale der Zelldifferenzierungen in normalem und pathologischem menschlichem Blut. Beiträge wurden nur von den ersten beiden zur Veröffentlichung eingereicht, die außerdem teilweise durch die verzögerte Drucklegung nicht mehr ihre ursprüngliche Aktualität besitzen (z. B. PATAKI über Monoaminoxydase-Latenz).

Neben der zusammenfassenden Darstellung der Robert-FEULGEN-Preisarbeit 1975 über die Beziehung der entero-endokrinen Zellen zur Serotoninsynthese sind vor allem die Übersichtsreferate des 2. Workshops von SCHNEIDER über theoretische Grundlagen und praktische Bedeutung der Enzymhemmung als Kontrollreaktionen und von GOSSRAU über Spezifitätsprobleme bei histochemischen Enzymnachweisen bedeutungsvoll. Letzteres enthält einen ganzen Katalog der Spezifitätsprobleme von dem zu untersuchenden Enzym selbst, über die vorbereitenden Maßnahmen zum Enzymnachweis, die Inkubation der Schnitte oder Blöcke, sowie die licht- bzw. elektronenmikroskopische Darstellung bis zur Nachbehandlung des inkubierten Gewebes. Hervorgehoben werden muß auch der Beitrag von INCZEDÉDY-MARCSEK und Mitarb. über dünnschichtchromatographische Extraktionsverfahren an Kryostatschnitten. Hier wird im Detail eine kombinierte histochemisch-chromatographische Methode an mehreren Beispielen erläutert und wie man damit entweder Lipide, freie Aminosäuren, Kohlenhydrate oder Steroide einzeln aus dem unfixierten oder fixierten Gewebe extrahieren, identifizieren und auch quantifizieren kann.

Als didaktisches Novum der Suppl.-Bd. werden die „Key-words" durch Fettdruck bei den Übersichtsreferaten hervorgehoben. Das Buch wird für Pathologen und Histochemiker gleichermaßen von Interesse sein.

D. W. R. BLEYL

IMMUNOLOGICAL ASPECTS OF FOODS. Herausgegeben von N. CATSIMPOOLAS. VIII und 400 Seiten, 102 Abb. und 32 Tab. The AVI Publishing Company, Inc. Westport (Connecticut) 1976, Preis 35,— $.

Das Buch gliedert sich in 4 Abschnitte. Im erten Teil („Food Proteins") werden Proteine aus Fleisch, Sojabohne, Gerste, Weizen, Erdnuß und Eiklar behandelt. Der 2. und 3. Abschnitt befaßt sich mit toxischen Substanzen aus Pflanzen und Tieren bzw. Bakterien und Viren, im einzelnen mit pflanzlichen Agglutininen und Proteaseinhibitoren, mit Toxinen aus Staphylokokken, Escherichia coli, Clostridien und aus Viren, die in Nahrungsmitteln enthalten sein können. In diesen 3 ersten Abschnitten werden die immunologischen Phänomene vornehmlich als methodische Hilfsmittel betrachtet. Ihre Anwendung eröffnet neue analytische Wege, und die Charakterisierung bestimmter Proteine gelingt überaupt erst mit immunchemischen Verfahren. Lediglich der 4. Abschnitt des Bandes („Food Allergy and Nutritional Immunology") befaßt sich mit immunologischen Erscheinungen, die beim Menschen infolge der Nahrungsaufnahme auftreten. Dazu gehören allergische Reaktionen, die von F. PERLMAN und speziell am Beispiel der Ölsaatenproteine von J. R. SPIES behandelt werden, sowie der Komplex Unterernährung und Immunität, von H. McFARLANE und M. R. C. PATH dargestellt. Der in diesem Thema gebotene Text ist freilich sehr knapp, eine genügend ausführliche Darstellung würde aber einen selbständigen Band füllen. Die Artikel sind verschiedentlich reich bebildert und durchweg mit umfangreichen Literaturverzeichnissen versehen. Der Band führt den Lebensmittelchemiker zweckmäßig und gewiß erfolgreich an immunologische Arbeitsmethoden heran.

H.J. ZUNFT

R. ZWILLING: IMMUNOLOGISCHES PRAKTIKUM. EINFÜHRUNG IN DIE METHODEN DER IMMUNCHEMIE. VIII und 77 Seiten, 21 Abb. Gustav Fischer Verlag, Stuttgart, New York 1977. Preis: 12,80 DM.

Der Autor beabsichtigt, den Studenten der Biologie, Biochemie oder Medizin eine Anleitung für ein etwa dreiwöchiges Praktikum in die Hand zu geben. Demgemäß sind die grundlegenden, einfachen Methoden der Immunologie zusammengestellt und erläutert, die sowohl die theoretischen Kenntnisse des Studenten festigen können, ihm aber auch die wirklich allgemein gebräuchlichen Arbeitstechniken vermitteln. Die großen Erfolge der Immunologie in den letzten Jahren beruhen ja großenteils auf den Vorzügen ihrer Methoden, der hohen Spezifität und der Empfindlichkeit, von denen Biochemie und Medizin zunehmend profitieren. Im einzelnen werden Anleitungen zu den Diffusionstechniken nach OUCHTERLONY, nach MANCINI und nach MERRILL, zur ein- und zweidimensionalen Immunelektrophorese, zur Komplementbindung, zur Immunfluoreszenz und zum Radioimmunoassay gegeben. Die klaren Anweisungen zum Einsatz von Geräten und Reagenzien sowie zur Versuchsdurchführung und -auswertung machen den Band als Laborhandbuch auch außerhalb des studentischen Praktikums wertvoll. H.-J. ZUNFT

Г. М. Уклистый и Н. П. Мартемьянова (G. M. UKLISTJ, und N. P. MARTEM'JANOVA): Микробиология рыбы и рыбных продуктов (MIKROBIOLOGIE VON FISCHEN UND FISCHERZEUGNISSEN). 143 Seiten, 43 Abb., 9 Tab., 57 Lit. Verlag Piščevaja Promyšlennost', Moskau 1976. Preis: 33 Kop.; 1,65 M.

Die vorliegende Broschüre ist als Lehrbuch der Mikrobiologie für Fachschulen der Fischkunde und Fischindustrie gedacht und fußt auf langjährigen Lehrerfahrungen. In 7 Kapiteln vermittelt es Grundkenntnisse über Mikroorganismen (Morphologie, Genetik, Systematik, Physiologie, insbesondere Fermentaktivität, Lebensbedingungen, Pathogenität und Toxine, Verbreitung). Im 8. Kapitel werden spezielle Fragen der mikrobiologischen Untersuchung in der Fischindustrie behandelt. Ausgehend von der Mikroflora des Fisches, wird auf Kontaminationsquellen und -wege sowie im Gewebe ablaufende, mikrobiologisch bedingte Prozesse eingegangen. Die zur mikrobiologischen Kontrolle bei der Herstellung der gebräuchlichsten Fischprodukte (Frischfisch, Filet, Salz-, Dörr-, Räucher- und marinierter Fisch, Kaviar, Präserven, Konserven, Fischmehl) durchzuführenden Untersuchungsschritte und Richtzahlen sind in Schemata zusammengestellt. Einbezogen sind Untersuchungen an Hilfs- und Zusatzstoffen sowie Fragen des Einflusses von Verpackung, Transport und Lagerung auf den mikrobiologischen Status. Insgesamt eine gut aufgebaute und umfassende Darstellung des Lehrstoffs. W. GOLDBACH

B. MALMGREN: EINFÜHRUNG IN DIE MIKROBIOLOGIE, 206 Seiten, 61 Abb., 8 Tab., Verlag F. K. Schattauer, Stuttgart—New York, 1976. Preis: 17,80 DM.

Mit dieser Übersetzung einer schwedischen Originalausgabe soll der sich auf mikrobiologischem Gebiet erstmals orientierende Leser — wie Oberschüler und Studenten — einen Überblick über die Mikrobiologie ganz allgemein, ihre Forschungsmethoden, aktuelle Probleme und Ergebnisse erhalten. Durch eine Auswahl interessanter elektronenmikroskopischer Aufnahmen versucht der Autor, neben den allgemeinen Grundlagen auch interessante neuere Erkenntnisse mikrobiologischer Forschung zu vermitteln. Allerdings ist ihm das nicht ausreichend gelungen, da das Buch in mehreren Details nicht mehr dem neuesten Stand der Forschung entspricht. Außerdem fällt im Vergleich zu anderen mikrobiologischen Büchern mit einführendem Charakter eine gewisse Unübersichtlichkeit auf.

A. QUEHL

А. С. Ратушный (A. S. RATUŠNYJ): Применение ферментов для обработки мяса (ANWENDUNG VON FERMENTEN IN DER FLEISCHVERARBEITUNG). 87 Seiten, 22 Abb., 17 Tab., 85 Lit. Verlag Piščevaja Promyšlennost', Moskva 1976. Preis: 31 Kop.; 1,55 M.

Ein Weg zur Intensivierung der technologischen Prozesse in der Fleischindustrie und zur Erhöhung der Qualität von Fleischprodukten besteht in der Anwendung von Proteasen. Die vorliegende Broschüre vermittelt hierzu einen guten Überblick. Nach Hinweis auf die Herkunft der Fermente (pflanzliche, tierische, mikrobielle) wird auf die proteolytische Aktivität und die sie beeinflussenden Faktoren (Milieu, Aktivatoren, Inhibitoren, Substrat, Temperatur) und die Arten der Anwendung (Injektion ins Blutgefäßsystem und Fleisch, Eintauchen in Lösungen, Bestreuen mit Pulver) eingegangen. Ein weiteres Kapitel behandelt Methoden zur Qualitätsbewertung von Fleisch nach Fermentanwendung (biologisch, biochemisch, instrumentell, organoleptisch). Der letzte Abschnitt befaßt sich mit den Forderungen nach toxikologischer Unbedenklichkeit der Fermentpräparate und nach deren Standardisierung. W. GOLDBACH

A. TÖPEL: CHEMIE UND PHYSIK DER MILCH. 472 Seiten, 138 Abb., 104 Tab. und 73 Übersichten. VEB Fachbuchverlag, Leipzig 1976. Preis: DDR 25,— M, Ausland 30,— M.

Zusammensetzung, Verhalten bei technologischen Verarbeitungsprozessen sowie ernährungsphysiologische Eigenschaften der Milch sind immer wieder Gegenstand wissenschaftlicher Untersuchungen und bedürfen einer zusammenfassenden Darstellung des gegenwärtigen Kenntnisstandes. Das vorliegende Werk ist daher zu begrüßen, zumal eine neuere deutschsprachige Monographie über diese Thematik nicht existiert. Im vorliegenden Buch behandelt der Autor das genannte Gebiet in 6 Kapiteln (Zusammensetzung der Milch; Bestandteile der Milch; Milch als polydisperses System; Physikalisch-chemische Eigenschaften; Beeinflussung durch Be- und Verarbeitung; Geschmacks- und Geruchsstoffe), wobei den Bestandteilen der Milch mit fast 200 Seiten der meiste Platz eingeräumt wird. Die einzelnen Sachverhalte werden ausführlich und durch eine gute Gliederung sowie anschauliche Abbildungen, Tabellen, Übersichten und Hervorhebungen in leicht faßlicher Form dargelegt. Dabei werden chemische, biochemische und physikalische Grundlagen jeweils zu Beginn der Abschnitte behandelt und dienen dem Verständnis bei Bearbeitungsvorgängen der Milch. Auf Wechselwirkungen der Milchbestandteile unter der Einwirkung verschiedener Einflußgrößen wird besonderer Wert gelegt.

Das Buch kann wegen seines hohen Informationsgehaltes zum angegebenen Thema Studenten und Fachleuten der Milchwirtschaft, Landwirtschaft sowie Lebensmittelchemie und -technologie empfohlen werden. U. BEHNKE

Н. Н. Пучеров (N. N. PUČEROV): Все о кофе (ALLES ÜBER KAFFEE). 87 Seiten. Verlag Naukova dumka, Kiev 1977. Preis: 14 Kop.

In populärwissenschaftlicher Form wird in dem vorliegenden Buch über das Vorkommen, die Bearbeitung, den Handel und über die Geschichte des Kaffees berichtet. Als Getränk wird Kaffee von medizinischen und chemischen Gesichtspunkten beleuchtet. Die Zusammensetzung der Kaffeearoma- und -geschmacksträger wird unter dem Gesichtspunkt dargelegt, daß dieses Buch nicht für Fachleute, sondern in erster Linie für interessierte Laien bestimmt ist. Das zeigt sich auch in der Rezepturensammlung, die ca. 1/4 des Buches umfaßt. Der Autor differenziert nicht nur zwischen heißen und kalten Getränken, sondern auch auf selbsthergestellte Konzentrate wird ebenso eingegangen, wie auf Cocktails, Liköre, Konditoreiwaren und kulinarische Erzeugnisse. Bei uns weniger verbreitete Kaffeezubereitungen im weitesten Sinn nehmen dabei einen breiten Raum ein. Zur Abrundung der Informationen über den Kaffee teilt der Autor noch einige Anekdoten aus der Kaffeehistorie mit und setzt damit erfolgreich seinen Weg fort, allgemeinverständlich alle Kaffeetrinker unterhaltsam zu informieren. R. BUSCH

G. MÜLLER: KLINISCHE BIOCHEMIE UND LABORATORIUMSDIAGNOSTIK. VEB Gustav Fischer Verlag, Jena 1978. 267 Seiten, 10 Tab., 5 Abb. Preis: 19,— M.

In straffer Form faßt der Autor das Gebiet der klinischen Biochemie und Laboratoriumsdiagnostik zusammen. Eine strenge Stoffauswahl erleichtert den Überblick. Der Verfasser verzichtet auf methodische Einzelheiten, da diese im DAB 7 (D. L.) für die DDR gesetzlich verbindlich erfaßt sind. In insgesamt 30 Kapiteln werden alle labordiagnostisch wesentlichen Komplexe erfaßt. Die einheitliche Gliederung garantiert eine schnelle Orientierung. Dem Autor ist es gelungen, die funktionellen Einheiten so darzustellen, daß der Zusammenhang zwischen Laboratoriumsdiagnostik, Pathophysiologie und Klinik deutlich hervorgehoben wird. Einführende Kapitel befassen sich ausführlich mit dem Probenmaterial, der Problematik der Referenzbereiche, der Qualitätskontrolle und den Möglichkeiten des Einsatzes der EDV. Dieses Buch stellt eine aktuelle Bereicherung der Arbeitsmaterialien für Chemiker und Ärzte in der Laboratoriumspraxis dar und ermöglicht dem behandelnden Arzt eine Übersicht des Fachgebietes. W. LÜDER

G. MÜLLER und R. KIESSING: EINFÜHRUNG IN DIE VERSUCHSTIERKUNDE. Band 1: ALLGEMEINE VERSUCHSTIERKUNDE. 204 Seiten, 11 Abb., 9 Tab. VEB Gustav Fischer Verlag, Jena 1977. Preis: 15,– M.

Der erste Band der „Einführung in die Versuchstierkunde", der als Leitfaden für tierexperimentell arbeitende Bereiche der Human-, Veterinärmedizin und Biologie gedacht ist, befaßt sich mit den theoretischen Grundlagen dieses Wissenskomplexes, der in den letzten Jahrzehnten an Bedeutung gewonnen hat. Ein historischer Abriß über die Verwendung von Tieren in der experimentellen Forschung zeigt die Entwicklung zu einer weitgehend eigenständigen Wissenschaft von den Versuchstieren. Dabei wird die Rolle der Labortiergenetik und Gnotobiologie besonders hervorgehoben. Der Überblick über Organisationen zur Förderung der Versuchstierkunde verdeutlicht, daß die Bereitstellung von Versuchstieren in der erforderlichen Qualität und Quantität international als wissenschaftliche Aufgabe angesehen wird, die eng mit der Lösung komplexer technologischer Probleme verbunden ist. Die Autoren legen in ihren Betrachtungen zum Ziel der Versuchstierwissenschaft großen Wert auf eine eindeutige Begründung und Definition versuchstierkundlicher Begriffe (z. B. Versuchstier, Laboratoriumstier) und unterscheiden zwei Formen von Tierversuchen: 1. Versuche, in denen Erkenntnisse über das Versuchstier als biologisches System angestrebt werden; 2. Versuche, in denen das Versuchstier als Modell für eine andere Art gilt (z. B. Modellierung menschlicher Krankheiten). Das Kapitel über Methoden der Versuchstierkunde ist gegliedert in genetische und gnotobiotische Methoden sowie Abschnitte über die definierte Umwelt der Versuchstiere, Beurteilung des Experiments und Qualität der Versuchstiere. Das Buch informiert außerdem über Anforderungen zur Qualifizierung der Wissenschaftler und über Ausbildung und Erziehung der wissenschaftlich-technischen Mitarbeiter, über Anwendungsgebiete der Versuchstierkunde und ökonomische Probleme im Zusammenhang mit der Durchführung von Tierexperimenten. H. J. LEWERENZ

VIII. INTERNATIONALER FRUCHTSAFT-KONGRESS, Meran 18.–21. 5. 1976, Kongreß-Bericht (14. Bericht der IFU). Zusammenstellung von H. J. BIELIG und H. TREPTOW. XLVI und 332 Seiten, 72 Abb., 63 Tab. Juris Druck & Verlag, Zürich 1977. Preis: 30,– sfrs.

Folgende Probleme wurden auf dem Fruchtsaftkongreß behandelt: Ökonomische und soziale Bedeutung der Fruchtsaftindustrie; Stand und Entwicklungstendenzen in der Technologie; Früchte und reine Fruchtsäfte für die menschliche Ernährung; chemische Zusammensetzung reiner Säfte; Fruchtsaftgewinnung durch Diffussion; Vorstudien zur kontinuierlichen Apfelsaftschönung; Einfluß verschiedener Schönungsmittel auf die Polyphenole in Kernobstsäften; Mikrobiologie von Fruchtsäften; Fruchtsaftnormen im Lichte technologischer und biochemischer Erkenntnisse; Analyse im Dienste der Qualitätskontrolle; Rückstände von Schädlingsbekämpfungsmitteln und Saftgewinnung; Beurteilung von natürlichem Fruchtaroma; französische Vorschriften und ihre Anwendung bei der Qualitätsbestimmung von Säften; Rohware für die Fruchtsaftherstellung – Produktion, Qualität, Preis; Image von Fruchtsäften; Verhältnisse zwischen Rohstoff- und Fruchtsaftherstellern; innere Qualität spanischer Orangen; Schutz und Information des Konsumenten in der Gesetzgebung der EWG; Fruchtsäfte im Wettbewerb sowie Produkt-Strategien für Fruchtsäfte. Die dargestellten Ergebnisse zeigen umfassend den wissenschaftlichen und technologischen Entwicklungsstand dieses zunehmend an Bedeutung gewinnenden Industriezweiges. Der angewandten Grundlagenforschung, der Einführung neuer Technologien, dem Einsatz verfeinerter Analysenverfahren, der Qualitätsüberwachung, aber auch dem Marketing wird viel Aufmerksamkeit geschenkt. G. DONGOWSKI

H. LEHMANN, E. RICHLOVSKY und B. WEIGEL: ALKOHOLFREIE GETRÄNKE. 100 Seiten, 8 Abb., 16 Tab. VEB Fachbuchverlag, Leipzig 1977. Preis: 5,80 M.

Die Verfasser stellen diesem Buch im Vorwort das Anliegen voraus, einen Überblick über das Gebiet der alkoholfreien Getränke geben zu wollen. Dieser Anspruch ist erfüllt worden. Darüber hinaus wird eine warenkundliche Abhandlung über Wasser, Obst- und Gemüsesäfte, Sirupe und Konzentrate sowie Spezialgetränke, u. a. Diabetikergetränke, kalorienreduzierte Getränke, gegeben. Die in der DDR gültigen Standards für Qualitätsbewertung, Transport und Lagerung werden jeweils angeführt. Die ernährungsphysiologische Betrachtung, die laut Vorwort ein Schwerpunkt sein soll, wird relativ unkritisch durchgeführt. Physiologische bzw. therapeutische Wirkungen werden meist überzeichnet, da die Aufnahmemenge in keinem Fall zur Frequenz und Gesamtkost in Relation gesetzt wird. Unklar ist die Sprachregelung dieses Aspektes.

In Tabelle 16 werden als physiologische Wirkungen erfrischend, nährend, anregend therapeutische Wirkung, geringer ernährungsphysiologischer Wert angegeben. Tomatensaft beispielsweise erhält mit 250 kcal/l das Prädikat nährend, während Kolagetränken und Fruchtsaftgetränken, die 300 kcal/l und mehr enthalten, nur ein erfrischender, anregender bzw. geringer ernährungsphysiologischer Wert bescheinigt wird. Der Genußwert wird trotz seiner eminenten Bedeutung vernachlässigt. Man vermißt eine Diskussion mindestens über die Rolle von Süße und Säure als Basis des Geschmacks und Erfrischungswertes jedes gesüßten Getränkes. Als Übersichtsinformation — besonders in warenkundlicher Hinsicht — schließt das Buch jedoch eine empfindliche Lücke. K. Hoppe

PEOPLE AND FOOD TOMORROW. Herausgegeben von D. Hollingsworth und E. Morse 173 Seiten, 9 Abb., 22 Tab., Applied Science Publ. Ltd., London 1976. Preis 20 $.

Das Buch enthält 15 Vorträge zu wissenschaftlichen, ökonomischen und sozialen Faktoren der Lebensmittelversorgung und Ernährung im letzten Viertel des 20. Jahrhunderts. Behandelt werden Qualität und Quantität der zur Verfügung stehenden Lebensmittel; Möglichkeiten der Produktionssteigerung; Bodenerosion und Wüstenbildung; Bodenverbrauch durch Verstädterung und Industrialisierung; Ernährungsbedarf, Bevölkerungszuwachs und steigende Bedürfnisse; Versorgung mit Energie, Eiweiß und Mikronährstoffen; die spezielle Situation in Großbritannien, Norwegen, Indien und in der VR China, die Bedeutung der Wissenschaft für die Weltlebensmittelproduktion (neue Technologien, neue Rohstoffe u. a.), Grenzen der Lebensmittelproduktion u. a. Aufgezeigt werden die Grenzen des Düngereinsatzes und der Verwendung neuer hochproduktiver Pflanzensorten. Für England wird aus Sorge um eine zu kurzsichtige Lebensmittelpolitik die Bildung eines Ministeriums für Lebensmittel (aus den bestehenden Ministerien für Landwirtschaft und Fischereiwesen, für Lebensmittelverarbeitung und -handel, für Ernährung, für EWG-Landwirtschaftspolitik und für Lebensmittelpreise) gefordert, damit soll eine ausgeglichene Gesamtplanung erreicht werden. In den Entwicklungsländern sei eine Abnahme des Bevölkerungszuwachses auch bei sich bessernden sozialökonomischen Verhältnissen nicht generell festzustellen.

Die Ernährungsprobleme in Entwicklungsländern werden in erster Linie auf die Armut zurückgeführt, nicht so sehr auf Bevölkerungswachstum oder Mangel an Lebensmitteln. Die früher behauptete Eiweißlücke stellt sich als ein sozialpolitisches Problem heraus, nämlich allen Bürgern genug der üblichen Lebensmittel zu sichern. Der Mangel an Vitamin A, Eisen (und Folsäure) sowie Jod ist von globaler, der von Thiamin, Niacin und Vitamin D von lokaler Bedeutung; Vitamin-C-Mangel spielt keine Rolle. Die wissenschaftlichen Möglichkeiten zur Steigerung der Lebensmittelproduktion zur Sicherung der globalen Ernährung werden positiv eingeschätzt.

In der Tierzucht wird der Zucht besonders ertragreicher, magerer Rinder (einschließlich Kreuzungen mit Yak oder Büffeln) Bedeutung beigemessen. Möglichkeiten werden in der verbesserten Nutzung von Abprodukten gesehen. In der Lebensmittelkonservierung wird ein Trend zu milderen Verfahren eingeschätzt.

Es gibt keine physiologische Notwendigkeit, den Eiweißverbrauch über durchschnittlich 25—30 g täglich anzuheben, sondern nur ein hedonistischer (lustbefriedigender) Drang nach tierischen Produkten wird behauptet. Die Bedeutung von Fleischsimulaten (aus Pflanzenprotein) liegt nicht in Entwicklungs-, sondern in Industrieländern, ihre Produktion erfordert eine relativ komplizierte und damit teure Technik. Einzellerproteine haben aus ökonomischen und toxikologischen Gründen für die menschliche Ernährung keine Bedeutung. Besondere Bedeutung kommt der Energiebilanzierung (Aufwand, Kosten, Nutzen) der landwirtschaftlichen Produktion zu.

Ein anregendes, inhaltsreiches Buch. H. Haenel

F. J. Stare und M. McWilliams: LIVING NUTRITION. 2. Aufl. X und 497 Seiten mit Abb. u. Tab. John Wiley and Sons, New York, Santa Barbara, London, Sydney, Toronto 1977. Preis: 8.70 £; 14.90 $.

Das vorliegende Buch ist vor allem als Lehrbuch und Nachschlagewerk für Studenten sowie für die allgemeine Ernährungsaufklärung gedacht.

Die Autoren verknüpfen biologische und soziale Aspekte im Sinne einer angewandten Ernährungslehre. Das Buch gliedert sich in 4 größere Kapitel, die durch zahlreiche Tabellen und Abbildungen illustriert sind: Sozialpsychologische Aspekte der Ernährung; Ernährung aus physiologischer Sicht; Ernährung in den einzelnen Lebensphasen; Angewandte Ernährung.

Im ersten Abschnitt findet der Leser eine kurze Darstellung der Welternährungssituation und der Nahrungsressourcen der Erde. Die Autoren lassen dabei zum Teil eine pessimistische Haltung erkennen. Im ersten Abschnitt findet sich außerdem eine Darstellung des Problems der Überernährung. Abschnitt 2 behandelt die Struktur und Funktion der einzelnen Stoffklassen der Nahrung: Kohlenhydrate, Lipide, Proteine, Wasser, Mineralien, Vitamine. Ernährungsempfehlungen für Schwangere und Stillende sowie für die einzelnen Entwicklungsphasen vom Säugling bis zum erwachsenen Menschen findet man in Abschnitt 3. Abschnitt 4 gibt Hinweise zur Ernährungspraxis in den USA.

Im Anhang des Buches befinden sich zahlreiche Tabellen und Übersichten zum ernährungsphysiologischen Wert von Nahrungsmitteln sowie Abbildungen von Vitamin- und Aminosäurestrukturen. Durch den großzügigen Druck und die Aufteilung in Unterabschnitte wirkt das Buch sehr übersichtlich und anschaulich.

I. Thiel

B. A. Kihlman: CAFFEINE AND CHROMOSOMES. 504 Seiten, 115 Abb., 44 Tab. Elsevier Scientific Publishing Company, Amsterdam, New York, Oxford 1977. Preis: 63,25 US $.

Coffein (1,3,7-Trimethylxanthin) stellt wegen seiner verschiedenartigen Wirkungen auf das genetische Material eine wichtige Verbindung für molekulargenetische Forschungen dar. Als Purin-Derivat ist es dem Adenin und Guanin verwandt, die Schlüsselverbindungen der als Träger und Übermittler der genetischen Information fungierenden Nucleinsäuren sind. Der Autor hat es übernommen, die umfangreiche Literatur über Coffein und seine Wirkungen unter genetischem Aspekt zu sichten und in einem ausführlichen Überblick zusammenzufassen.

Der erste Teil des Buches wird mit einer historischen Betrachtung der Entdeckung von Coffein und der Entwicklung der Strukturformel eingeleitet. Es folgen Ausführungen über Vorkommen und Biosynthese in Pflanzen, Metabolismus und pharmakologische Wirkungen sowie über coffeinhaltige Getränke.

Der zweite Teil, der die Überschrift „Chromosomen" trägt, stellt praktisch eine Einführung in die Molekulargenetik dar. Betrachtet werden: Chemie, Struktur und Replikation der Chromosomen; Struktur, Replikation, Schädigung und Erneuerung der DNS; Mutationen und Chromosomenaberrationen.

Die Wirkungen von Coffein und verwandten Verbindungen auf diese Systeme behandelt der dritte Teil, der mit einem Kapitel zur Risikobewertung der Verbindung abschließt. Darin wird festgestellt, daß Coffein in den Mengen, die der Mensch bei normalem Verbrauch coffeinhaltiger Getränke und medizinischer Präparate aufnimmt, keine mutagenen, chromosomenschädigenden, carcinogenen oder teratogenen Wirkungen hat. Unter Hinweis auf neuere Ergebnisse empfiehlt der Autor jedoch, einen starken Kaffeekonsum in den frühen Phasen einer Schwangerschaft zu vermeiden.

H. J. Lewerenz

PHENOLIC, SULFUR, AND NITROGEN COMPOUNDS IN FOOD FLAVORS. Herausgegeben von G. Charalambous und I. Katz, 215 Seiten. 75 Abb., 34 Tab. American Chemical Society, Washington 1976. Preis: 17,75 $.

Das Buch ist der Band 26 der „ACS Symposium Series" und beinhaltet 12 Vorträge eines von der Division of Agricultural and Food Chemistry veranstalteten Symposiums auf dem 170. Treffen der American Chemical Society 1975 in Chicago. Die Titel der Vorträge lauten: Rolle von Flavonen und verwandten Verbindungen bei der Verzögerung fett-oxydativer Flavorveränderungen in Lebensmitteln (D. E. Pratt); Beitrag polyphenolischer Verbindungen zum Teegeschmack (G. W. Sanderson u. a.); Weinflavor und phenolische Substanzen (V. L. Singleton und A. C. Noble); Überwachung und Kontrolle phenolischen Geschmacks und Geruchs in Wasser zur Verhinderung ihrer

Einflüsse auf Geschmack und Flavor von Lebensmitteln (B. F. WILLEY); Simultaner Nachweis von N- und S-haltigen Aromastoffen (D. A. WITHYCOMBE u. a.); Aromavorläufer in Lebensmitteln (L. SCHUTTE); Reaktionsprodukte von α-Dicarbonylverbindungen, Aldehyden, Sulfid und Ammoniak (H. J. TAKKEN); Nichtenzymatische Transaminierung ungesättigter Carbonyle: eine generelle Quelle für N-haltige Aromastoffe in Lebensmitteln (G. P. RIZZI); Identifizierung und Flavoreigenschaften einiger 3-Oxazoline und 3-Thiazoline aus gekochtem Rindfleisch (C. J. MUSSINAN u. a.); Nichtflüchtige N- und S-Verbindungen in roten Fleischarten und ihre Beziehungen zu Flavor und Geschmack (A. F. MABROUK); In 3-Stellung mit S substituierte Furane (W. J. EVERS u. a.); Neurale Geschmackserwiderung von N-Verbindungen bei Katzen (J. C. BOCEREAU u. a.). Die Vorträge geben einen repräsentativen Überblick über den in den letzten Jahren sprunghaft angestiegenen Wissensstand auf dem Gebiet dieser wichtigen Gruppe von Aromastoffen.

W. RÖDEL

А. Н. Зайдель, Г. В. Островская и Ю. И. Островский (A. N. ZAJDEL', G. W. OSTROWSKAJA und J. I. OSTROWSKIJ): Техника и практика спектроскопии (DIE TECHNIK UND PRAXIS DER SPEKTROSKOPIE). 2. Aufl., 392 Seiten, 362 Abb., 25 Tab. Verlag Nauka, Moskau 1976. Preis: 2 Rub. 40 Kop.; 12,— M.

In diesem Band der Serie „Physik und Technik der Spektralanalyse" werden die theoretischen Grundlagen des Aufbaus und der Funktionsweise von Spektralanalysengeräten, die im Wellenlängenbereich von 200 bis 1000 nm arbeiten, sehr ausführlich abgehandelt. Im einzelnen vermitteln die 15 Kapitel Grundkenntnisse über Prismen und Gitter, Klassifizierungen und Charakteristiken der Spektralgeräte, Lichtquellen, Focussierungs- und Filtersysteme, Energie- und Wellenlängenmessungen, Auflösungsvermögen und Dispersion. Die Weiterentwicklung der spektroskopischen Methoden in den letzten Jahren kommt in dieser 2. überarbeiteten und ergänzten Auflage u. a. dadurch zum Ausdruck, daß in einigen Kapiteln die Laserstrahlenanwendung den entsprechenden Raum einnimmt.

Das in erster Linie für den Studenten der allgemeinen und angewandten Spektroskopie geschriebene Buch ist sicherlich keine Fundgrube für den praktisch tätigen Analytiker, da die Kapitel ausschließlich auf die gerätetechnische Seite und nur in einigen Ausnahmen auf die Spektroskopie von Elementen ausgerichtet sind. Ungeachtet dessen stellen die dargelegten theoretischen Grundlagen der Aufbauelemente von Spektralgeräten und der methodischen Handhabung in ihrer Ausführlichkeit und Fülle hohe Anforderungen an den interessierten Leser.

R. SCHRÖDTER

Б. И. Анваер и Ю. С. Другов (B. I. ANWAER und Ju. S. DRUGOW): Газовая хроматография неорганических веществ. (DIE GASCHROMATOGRAPHIE ANORGANISCHER STOFFE). 239 Seiten, zahlr. Abb. und Tab., Verlag Chemie, Moskau 1976. Preis: 4,35 M.

Die gaschromatographische Analyse von Gasen, aggressiven Stoffen, Wasser, Metallbestandteilen, metallorganischen Verbindungen, Anionen und zur Klärung physikochemischer Prozesse ist eine besonders elegante Methode. In den letzten Jahren hat insbesondere die Anwendung der Gaschromatographie in der Mineralstofforschung neue analytische Möglichkeiten eröffnet.

Übersichtlich durch Tabellen und Chromatogramme ergänzt, geben die Autoren eine stark gedrängte Zusammenfassung des Arbeitsgebietes. In den nach Verbindungsarten und Elementen geordneten Kapiteln des Werkes findet sich der Leser auch ohne Stichwortregister zurecht.

Zahlreiche Hinweise ermöglichen den Zugang zur sowjetischen, angelsächsischen und japanischen Literatur.

R. M. MACHOLZ

S. LEWIN: VITAMIN C — ITS MOLECULAR BIOLOGY AND MEDICAL POTENTIAL. 231 Seiten, 23 Abb., 10 Tab., zahlreiche Formelschemata. Academic Press, London, New York, San Francisco 1976. Preis: 7,80 £.

Seit Linus PAULING 1970 mit seinem Buch „Vitamin C and the Common Cold" weltweit Aufsehen erregte, ist der Meinungsstreit über die Notwendigkeit oder Nützlichkeit von „Mega-Aufnahmen" an Vitamin C nicht abgerissen. Im Unterschied zu den bisherigen Auslassungen, in denen hohe Zufuhrempfehlungen aus vergleichenden biologischen Betrachtungen, evolutionärer Sicht und pharmakologischer Erfahrung abgeleitet worden sind, wird im vorliegenden Buch von S. LEWIN versucht, sie auf molekularbiologischer und biochemischer Ebene zu begründen. In 3 Teilen und 9 Kapiteln wird unter Bezug auf 466 Literaturstellen und eigene Untersuchungsergebnisse, reich untergliedert, auf die chemische und biochemische Reaktivität des Ascorbatsystems, dessen Biosynthese, Stoffwechsel und biologische Wirkungen sowie auf medizinische und genetische Aspekte des Ascorbinsäurebedarfs eingegangen. Der modus operandi wird zum einen direkt auf charakteristische physikochemische Eigenschaften (ionisierter Zustand, Oxydations-Reduktions-Vermögen, Herabsetzung der Oberflächenspannung, Beteiligung an Wasserstoffbrücken-Bindungen) zurückgeführt. Zum anderen soll er indirekt auf der Beeinflussung von Enzymaktivitäten (z. B. bei der Kollagen- und Antikörperbildung), der Einbeziehung in die Bildung von Hormonen wie Adrenalin, Noradrenalin und Serotonin, der Einwirkung auf die Enzymbiosynthese, der Entgiftung endogener und exogener toxischer Stoffe (z. B. von Adrenochrom, Barbituraten oder Nitrosaminen), einer gewissen Antihistaminaktivität sowie letzten Endes und insbesondere auf einer Regulierung der Blut- und Gewebespiegel an c-AMP und c-GMP und damit einer ganzen Reihe von Stoffwechselprozessen und physiologischen Reaktionen beruhen. Eine Erhöhung dieser Spiegel wird von der Aktivierung der Adenylcyclase über eine Förderung der Synthese von Adrenalin und der Verhinderung von dessen Oxydation zu Adrenochrom sowie einer Herabsetzung der Phosphodiesteraseaktivität infolge Besetzung der aktiven Zentren hergeleitet. Da sich die zellulären c-AMP-Konzentrationen im Bereich von 10^{-6} bis 10^{-4} M bewegen, müssen die Ascorbatspiegel vergleichsweise hoch sein und im Blutserum durchschnittlich bei 2 mg/100 ml liegen. Um dies zu erreichen, werden tägliche Zufuhren von 0,5 bis 20 g empfohlen. Die große Schwankungsbreite des individuellen Bedarfs sowie widersprüchliche Untersuchungsergebnisse werden mit unterschiedlicher Nettoaufnahme (Oxydation und Delaktonisierung vor Übergang in den Blutstrom), Belastung (körperliche und seelische Belastungen, Erkältung, Trauma, Schock u. ä.) und Biosynthese zu erklären versucht. Die mit den durch die üblicherweise empfohlenen geringen Tagesdosen erreichbare Verhinderung oder Beseitigung von Skorbut zielt nach Auffassung des Autors lediglich auf ein Symptom ausgeprägten Ascorbinsäuremangels. Alles in allem: ein Buch, das zur Auseinandersetzung reizt und eine Fülle von Anregungen für die Forschung vermittelt.

B. GASSMANN

PROTEIN METABOLISM AND NUTRITION. Herausgegeben von D. J. A. COLE, K. N. BOORMAN, P. J. BUTTERY, D. LEWIS, R. J. NEALE und H. SWAN, 515 Seiten, 101 Abb., 124 Tab. Butterworths, London 1976. Preis: 19,20 £.

Der Band stellt eine Sammlung der 27 Vorträge dar, die 1974 beim „1. Symposium über Proteinstoffwechsel und Ernährung" der European Association for Animal Production in Nottingham gehalten wurden. Das Spektrum der Beiträge reicht von der allgemeinen theoretischen Abhandlung des gegenwärtigen Erkenntnisstandes auf Teilgebieten der Bereiche Ernährung und Proteinstoffwechsel bis zur wissenschaftlichen Bearbeitung praktischer Probleme der Nutztierfütterung. Da die Autoren nicht ausschließlich auf dem Gebiet der Tierernährung tätig sind, wendet sich eine ganze Reihe von Beiträgen auch an den großen Kreis derer, die biochemisch oder physiologisch an Fragen der Eiweißernährung des Menschen interessiert sind. Das gilt z. B. für folgende Artikel:

Eukaryote Proteinsynthese und ihre Kontrolle (H. N. MUNRO), Aminosäureversorgung und Proteinsynthese in tierischen Zellen (M. J. CLEMENS und V. M. PAIN), Hormonelle Kontrolle des Proteinstoffwechsels (K. L. MANCHESTER), Proteinumsatz (D. J. MILLWARD u. a.), Aminosäuretransport (B. G. MUNCK), Proteinverdauung und -absorption (A. RERAT, T. CORRING und J. P. LAPLACE), Aminosäureverfügbarkeit (H. ERBERSDOBLER), Aminosäuren als Energiequelle (D. B. LINDSAY), Energetischer Nutzeffekt des Aminosäurestoffwechsels (P. J. BUTTERY und K. N. BOORMAN), Der Energieaufwand für den Proteinansatz (J. KIELANOWSKI), Indirekte Messungen zur Proteinbewertung (B. O. EGGUM), Nahrungseffekte und Aminosäuren in Geweben (R. PION), Ernährungs- und Stoffwechselwirkungen von Aminosäureimbalancen (Q. R. ROGERS)

Mit hoher Informationsdichte werden Einführung in die Gesamtproblematik und Überblick über den internationalen Stand auf dem behandelten Teilgebiet der Ernährung geboten. Die Ergänzung der zahlreich zitierten Primärliteratur bis 1975 verleiht diesem empfehlenswerten Buch große Aktualität.

H. PRZYBILSKI

А. А. Покровский и Л. П. Крыстев (A. A. POKROVSKIJ und L. P. KRYSTEV): Печень, лизосомы и питание (LEBER, LYSOSOME UND ERNÄHRUNG). 208 Seiten, 21 Tab., 64 Abb. Verlag der Bulgarischen Akademie der Wissenschaften, Sofia 1977. Preis: 3.50 Lewa.

In drei mehr einleitenden, klar gegliederten Abschnitten werden sowohl die derzeitigen Ansichten über die morphologisch-funktionellen Besonderheiten der Zellen der Leber als auch einige grundlegende metabolische Prozesse in der Leber behandelt. Hervorgehoben wird die morphologisch-funktionelle Einheit der Lysosome, was auch besonders bei der Besprechung der Rolle des enzymatischen Komplexes der Lysosome hervortritt. Auf Grund eigener detaillierter Untersuchungen und vorliegender Literatur (901 Zitate) wird auf die engen Beziehungen zwischen dem strukturellen Aufbau der Lysosome und den Verdauungsprozessen im Organismus hingewiesen. Unter anderem wird auch auf die Probleme des Hungerns in biomedizinischer Hinsicht eingegangen. Eine vollwertige Ernährung der Menschheit erscheint als ein noch lange nicht gelöstes Problem. Die vorliegende Thematik spricht vor allen Dingen Ernährungsspezialisten, Biochemiker und Pathologen an, es werden aber auch allgemeinmedizinische und Fragen rein biologischen Charakters berührt. M. ULMANN

WHO-IARC MONOGRAPHS ON THE EVALUATION OF CARCINOGENIC RISK OF CHEMICALS TO MAN. VOL. 13: SOME MISCELLANEOUS PHARMACEUTICAL SUBSTANCES. 255 Seiten. International Agency for Research on Cancer, Lyon 1977. Preis: 30,— sfrs.; 12.00 US $.

Im Band 13 werden 22 Pharmaka hinsichtlich einer möglichen kanzerogenen Wirkung beurteilt. Einleitend wird auf eine mögliche endogene Bildung kanzerogener Nitrosoderivate von Pharmaka mit sekundären und tertiären Aminogruppen im Gestrointestinaltrakt des Menschen hingewiesen.

Folgende Pharmaka konnten nicht beurteilt werden, weil die Unterlagen unzureichend waren: Acetylsalicylsäure, Amobarbital, Chlorpromazin, Diphenylthiohydantoin, LSD, Nitroxolin, Natriumpentobarbital, Prednison, Pyrazinamid, Rifampicin und Spironolacton. Folgende Pharmaka werden tierexperimentell als kanzerogen beurteilt: Aurothioglucose, Diazepam, Oxazepam, Dithranol, Ethionamid, Hycanthonmesylat, Metronidazol, Nirodazol, der Metabolit des Phenacetins (Hydroxyphenacetin), Phenobarbital, Phenotoin, Pronetalolhydrochlorid, Pyrimethamin. Bei Acriflavinchlorid, Chlorequin, 8-Hydroxychinolin und Oxymetholon ist eine Beurteilung der kanzerogenen Wirkung z. Z. nicht möglich, weil die experimentellen Versuchsanordnungen als nicht ausreichend eingeschätzt wurden. Eine Beziehung zwischen Pharmakagabe und Krebsentstehung beim Menschen ist bei Phenacetin-Abusus und Phenotoin wahrscheinlich, bei Oxymetholon, Phenobarbital und Phenylbutazon und Oxyphenbutazon nicht ausgeschlossen.

Die einführenden Kapitel behandeln u. a. Zweck der Monographien, Gesichtspunkte für die Beurteilung, Terminologie, Dosis-Wirkungsbeziehungen bei Karzinogenen, Extrapolation vom Versuchstier auf den Menschen und Auswahl der hier diskutierten Substanzen. Jede als kanzerogen suspekte Substanz wird nach einem bereits beschriebenen Schema abgehandelt, die zitierte Literatur und die übersichtliche Gliederung ermöglichen eine einheitliche Beurteilung der Noxen und stellen eine Arbeitsgrundlage für jeden auf diesem Gebiet Tätigen dar. W. FRITZ

DOCUMENTA GEIGY, WISSENSCHAFTLICHE TABELLEN SUPPLEMENTUM II: INFEKTIONSKRANKHEITEN UND IHRE ERREGER, Hrsg.: Ciba — Geigy AG Basel. Redaktion: K. DIEM und C. LENTNER unter Mitarbeit von J. G. BAER, E. BERGER, H. BRODHAGE, M. FERNEX, L. P. GARROD, R. GEIGY, O. GSELL, M. KAUFFMANN, M. KOCH, H. P. R. SEELIGER, Ciba — Geigy AG, Basel 1967, Unveränderter Nachdruck 1972, 162 Seiten.

Übersichtlichkeit, Prägnanz und Kürze der Darstellung des Wesentlichen kennzeichnen die von allen praktisch tätigen Ärzten geschätzten wissenschaftlichen Tabellen der Documenta Geigy. In diesem Band der Infektionskrankheiten werden alle derzeit im mitteleuropäischen Raum auftretenden Infektionskrankheiten erfaßt, wobei jeweils ätiologische, pathophysiologische, klinische und therapeutische Hinweise gegeben werden. Ausgehend von einem Abschnitt über Häufigkeit von Infektionskrankheiten, werden in weiteren Kapiteln Infektionen durch Bakterien, Viren, Pilze, Protozoen und Würmer in kurzen Texten abgehandelt und durch informative Tabellen bzw. Abbildungen ergänzt.

Hinweise auf Entnahme und Versand von Untersuchungsmaterial, über Einteilung, Herkunft, Pharmakologie und therapeutischen Einsatz von Antibiotika sowie eine tabellarische Übersicht internationaler biologischer Standard- und Referenz-Präparate beschließen diesen Band.

K. Vetter

H. J. Raderecht: PATHOBIOCHEMIE DES LIPIDSTOFFWECHSELS. 166 Seiten, 19 Abb., 8 Tab. VEB Verlag Volk und Gesundheit, Berlin 1977. Preis: 21,10 M.

Der zunehmenden Aufmerksamkeit, die dem Lipidstoffwechsel geschenkt wird, Rechnung tragend, gibt der Autor in übersichtlicher und geraffter Form einen Überblick über das gegenwärtig gesicherte Wissen über den Lipidstoffwechsel bei besonderer Berücksichtigung der pathologischen Veränderungen. Einleitend werden Verdauung und Resorption der Nahrungsfette sowie das Plasmalipidsystem hinsichtlich seiner Zusammensetzung und Funktion dargestellt. Unter dem Aspekt von endogener Synthese und Abbau wird der Stoffwechsel von Fettsäuren, Triglyceriden, Phospholipiden und Cholesterin behandelt, wobei die Hormoneinflüsse auf den Fettstoffwechsel besonders herausgestellt sind. Dem Fettgewebe als Speicherorgan für Energiereserven ist ein gesondertes Kapitel gewidmet, um seine besondere Rolle im Lipidstoffwechsel des Organismus und bei der Entwicklung der Adipositas zu unterstreichen. In systematisch gegliederter Form werden dann die Lipopathien wie Hyperlipidämien und Lipidosen hinsichtlich Symptomatik und Stoffwechsel beschrieben, ein Diagnoseschema für Hyperlipidämien sowie eine Darstellung aktueller Probleme des Lipidstoffwechsels von Zellmembranen (Erythrozytenmembran- und Oberflächenschicht der Lungenalveolen) schließt die gelungene Monographie ab. Ein umfangreicher Literaturanhang verweist auf vertiefende Publikationen. Die als Lehrmaterial konzipierte Darstellung des Lipidstoffwechsels wird besonders den Laboratoriumswissenschaftler und Kliniker zur Vertiefung des theoretischen Wissens ansprechen, aber auch in der Aus- und Weiterbildung einen besonderen Platz einnehmen.

L. Aust

TASCHENBUCH DER PATHOPHYSIOLOGIE FÜR MEDIZINER UND ERNÄHRUNGSWISSENSCHAFTLER. Bd. 2. Herausgegeben von H. J. Holtmeier. 448 Seiten. Gustav Fischer, Stuttgart 1976. Preis: 23,80 DM.

Auch der 2. Band dieses instruktiven Taschenbuches wird der Absicht des Herausgebers gerecht, Grundlagen der Pathophysiologie in unmittelbarer Beziehung zu Nahrungs- und Ernährungseinflüssen darzustellen. Folgende Organe bzw. Organsysteme werden unter dem Aspekt pathophysiologischer Veränderungen behandelt: Blut, Leber, Galle und Gallenwege, Pankreas, Schilddrüse und im Kapitel „Endokrinologie" Hypothalamus und Hypophyse sowie Nebenniere. Auf bestimmte Funktionen einiger dieser Organe nehmen auch die Beiträge Bezug, die sich generell mit Störungen von Verdauung und Resorption, allgemeinem Stoffwechsel und Kohlenhydratstoffwechsel (Diabetes mellitus) befassen. Dabei ist das Bemühen der Autoren erkennbar, Überschneidungen weitgehend zu vermeiden. Weitere Kapitel gelten der Rolle calciumregulierender Hormone, den Vitaminen, den Spurenelementen und dem Mineral- und Wasserhaushalt im Organismus und damit zusammenhängenden pathophysiologischen Problemen. Der zweifellos interessante Überblick über Auswirkungen von Pestiziden auf das Ökosystem fällt aus dem Rahmen einer pathophysiologischen Betrachtungsweise. Im Zusammenhang mit den Ausführungen über die pathophysiologischen Wirkungen von Pflanzenschutz- und Schädlingsbekämpfungsmitteln wird der Leser auch über den biologischen Landbau informiert, was sich in einem Pathophysiologiebuch ebenfalls recht ungewöhnlich ausnimmt.

Dem Kapitel „Pathologische Probleme der Pharmakologie und Toxikologie der Ernährung" liegt folgende Stoffauswahl zugrunde: 1. Natürlicherweise in pflanzlichen oder tierischen Produkten vorkommende Wirkstoffe; 2. Kontamination von Lebensmitteln mit Bakterien, Pilzen oder Viren; 3. Lebensmittelzusatzstoffe; 4. Kontamination von Lebensmitteln mit Pestiziden und Schwermetallen.

Das Buch schließt mit einem Beitrag über die schädlichen Wirkungen des Nicotins und Tabellen über die Umrechnungsfaktoren für Elektrolyte sowie die Nährwerte der wichtigsten Nahrungsmittel.

H. J. Lewerenz

ATHEROSCLEROSIS — III. Proceedings of the Third International Symposium on Atherosclerosis — Berlin (West), October 24—28th, 1973. Herausgegeben von G. SCHETTLER u. A. WEIZEL. XXXV und 1034 Seiten, 349 Abb., 222 Tab. Springer-Verlag Berlin, Heidelberg, New York 1974. Preis: 32 $.

Die Ergebnisse des Symposiums werden sowohl in Form ausführlicher Übersichten als auch von Kurzreferaten mitgeteilt. Eine große Anzahl sehr instruktiver Abb. und Tab. erläutern den Text wirkungsvoll. Sowohl zu den Übersichten als auch zu Komplexthemen werden die Diskussionen angeführt. Ebenso enthält die Veröffentlichung Zusammenfassungen zu den auf der Tagung durchgeführten Workshops. Ein umfangreiches Literaturverzeichnis nimmt 80 Seiten ein. Eine Liste der Autoren und ihrer Anschriften vervollständigt die Informationen.

In 29 Kapiteln wird zu im wesentlichen 4 Komplexen Stellung genommen. Einen ersten Schwerpunkt bilden Fragen der Pathogenese der atherosklerotischen Veränderungen der Gefäßwand. Dabei werden abgehandelt: die Art der Läsionen, der Stoffwechsel der Gefäßwand (Lipoproteine, Lipide, Enzyme, allgemeiner Stoffwechsel, kontraktile Proteine), Permeabilitätsveränderungen, Thrombogenese und Fibrinolyse. Es folgt ein Komplex, der sich mit tierexperimentellen Modellen und dem Lipid-, besonders Lipoproteinstoffwechsel von Versuchstieren befaßt. Einen weiteren Schwerpunkt bilden die Kapitel, die vorwiegend dem Lipidstoffwechsel bei HLP (Mensch) gewidmet sind (Genetik, Epidemiologie, Plasmalipid- und Lipoproteinstoffwechsel, lipolytische Enzyme, Faktoren, die die HLP/Atherosklerose fördern). In einem 4. Komplex wird auf Risikofaktoren, Fragen der Prävention und der nutriven und medikamentösen Therapie (sowie kurz auch chirurgische Therapie) eingegangen.

Die Veröffentlichung ist eine wertvolle Fundquelle für alle angeschnittenen Fragen der Atherosklerose, gibt eine breitgefächerte Übersicht zum Stand der Kenntnisse und (in Verbindung mit den vorher erschienenen Kongreßberichten Atherosclerosis I und II) zu den erzielten Fortschritten in Theorie und Praxis. R. NOACK

J. L. van LANCKER: MOLECULAR AND CELLULAR MECHANISMS IN DISEASE. Bd. 1: XV und 603 Seiten, 266 Abb.; Bd. 2: VII und 1116 Seiten, 145 Abb. Springer-Verlag Berlin, Heidelberg, New York 1976. Preis insges.: 148,50 $.

Das von einem erfahrenen Hochschullehrer (Pathologe, Pathobiochemiker) verfaßte Werk gibt eine umfangreiche, z. T. sehr detaillierte, anspruchsvolle und anregende Übersicht über molekulare und zelluläre Mechanismen bei Erkrankungen.

Im 1. Band werden auf der Grundlage moderner biochemischer Kenntnisse und Entwicklungen sehr gründlich folgende Aspekte behandelt: zelluläre Energiebereitstellung, Zellspezifität (u. a. genetischer Code, Proteinsynthese), angeborene Stoffwechselstörungen, Fehlernährung (exogen oder endogen bedingt), Bio- und Pathobiochemie von Calcium, Eisen, Gallenpigmenten, Hormonen, Elektrolyten und Körperflüssigkeiten sowie der Blutgerinnung. Mit z. T. stärkerer morphologischer Ausrichtung enthält der 2. Band folgende Kapitel: Zelltod und Degeneration, Blutlipide und Arteriosklerose, Strahlenschäden, Entzündung, Immunpathologie, Regeneration, Hypertrophie und Wundheilung, Krebs.

Durch kluge Auswahl wesentlicher Fakten konnte ein Übersichtswerk vorgelegt werden, in dem Zusammenhänge zwischen biochemischen und morphologischen Charakteristika der normalen und der Pathobiologie dargelegt werden. Auf offene Fragen wird mehrfach verwiesen. Der Text wird durch zahlreiche informative Abbildungen erläutert. Die zitierte Literatur (bis 1974) enthält vor allem zusammenfassende Darstellungen, aber auch wichtige Einzelarbeiten. Die auf zahlreichen Gebieten noch bestehenden Wissenslücken bedingten, daß in einigen Unterkapiteln eine Beschränkung auf ausgewählte Aspekte erfolgte (z. B. Adipositas). Vereinzelt erscheinen Einzelbefunde gegenüber der Darstellung komplexer Stoffwechselveränderungen zu sehr betont (z. B. Malnutrition). Stellenweise ist eine Aktualisierung wünschenswert (z. B. Malabsorption und Dünndarmenzyme, frühkindliche Mangelernährung und deren Folgen). Unabhängig davon dürfte jedoch dieses Werk von großem Nutzen und sehr anregend für alle an der Thematik Interessierten sein. R. NOACK

FETTEMULSIONEN IN DER PARENTERALEN ERNÄHRUNG. Herausgegeben von A. WRETLIND, R. FREY, K. EYRICH und H. MAKOWSKI. 222 Seiten, 95 Abb. Springer-Verlag Berlin, Heidelberg, New York 1977. Preis: 48,— DM.

Der vorliegende Band 103 aus der Reihe „Anaesthesiologie und Wiederbelebung" enthält Vorträge sowie Diskussionsbeiträge anläßlich eines Symposiums im Juni 1976 in Stockholm mit der Zielstellung, dem praktisch tätigen Kliniker einen Leitfaden für seine tägliche Arbeit an die Hand zu geben. Von zahlreichen Spezialisten wird der Stand der Kenntnisse zu ausgewählten Problemen auf dem weitgefächerten Gebiet der parenteralen Ernährung vorgetragen. Wenn auch allein schon durch Titelwahl des Bandes sowie zahlreiche spezielle Vorträge auf die besondere Bedeutung der Fettemulsionen innerhalb des Symposiums und damit im Bereich der parenteralen Ernährungstherapie hingewiesen wird, so befassen sich darüber hinaus weitere Beiträge mit der Rolle der Kohlenhydrate und Aminosäuren im Rahmen dieses speziellen Ernährungsregimes. Des weiteren wird über Erfahrungen mit dieser Ernährungsform bei verschiedenen Krankheiten berichtet. Schließlich wird dargelegt, daß mit den heute zur Verfügung stehenden Präparaten eine vollständige parenterale Ernährung monatelang möglich ist.

Am Ende eines jeden Vortrages sind zur Stoffvertiefung zahlreiche Literaturstellen angefügt, und am Schluß des Bandes ermöglicht ein Sachwortverzeichnis die schnelle Auffindung von gezielten Informationen. Das Buch vermittelt eine Vielzahl von Erfahrungen und Empfehlungen und bietet eine gute Orientierungshilfe. J. KROLL

Биохимия гормонов и гормональной регуляции (BIOCHEMIE DER HORMONE UND DER HORMONELLEN REGULATION). 380 Seiten, 67 Abb., 14 Tab. Verlag Nauka, Moskau 1976. Preis: 1,82 Rbl.; 9,10 M.

Die von einem sowjetischen Autorenkollektiv unter der Leitung von N. A. JUDAEV geschriebene Monographie behandelt den neueren Stand der Biochemie der Hormone und der hormonellen Regulation von Stoffwechselprozessen auf molekularer und zellulärer Ebene. Im ersten Teil des Buches werden Struktur und Wirkungsweise der Peptid- und Proteinhormone des Hypothalamus, der Hypophyse, der Bauchspeicheldrüse sowie des Parathormons und des Kalzitonins beschrieben. Des weiteren folgt ein Kapitel zu den Steroidhormonen, in dem zunächst auf das Cholesterin als Vorläufer dieser Hormonklasse und danach im Einzelnen auf Corticosteroide, Aldosteron und Sexualhormone eingegangen wird. Das 3. Kapitel behandelt Struktur, Verbreitung und Gehalt im Organismus, Biosynthese, Umwandlungen sowie die biologische Wirkungsweise der Prostaglandine. Wertvoll ist zweifellos das letzte Kapitel, in dem die neuen Erkenntnisse zu den Wirkungsmechanismen der Hormone zusammengefaßt wurden. Zahlreiche Literaturangaben, zum großen Anteil von nach 1970 bis teilweise 1974, vervollständigen die einzelnen Kapitel.

Alle gegenwärtig bekannten Hormone wurden allerdings nicht berücksichtigt. So sind z. B. Thyroxin und Trijodthyronin sowie Adrenalin nicht besprochen worden. Ein Sachwortverzeichnis ist ebenfalls nicht vorhanden.

Auf Grund der Aktualität des für Biochemiker und Mediziner gut verständlich geschriebenen Buches und eines Defizits qualifizierterer Literatur zu den aktuellen Problemen der hormonellen Regulation erscheint eine Übersetzung ins Deutsche wünschenswert. K. J. PETZKE

Autorenkollektiv: LEBENSMITTEL FÜR DIE GESUNDE ERNÄHRUNG. EINE WARENKUNDE ÜBER LEBENSMITTEL FÜR DIE DIÄTETISCHE ERNÄHRUNG. 248 Seiten, 15 teils farbige Abb., 53 Tab. VEB Fachbuchverlag, Leipzig 1977. Preis: 10,80 M.

Das Sortiment an neuen, für bestimmte Konsumentengruppen geschaffenen Lebensmitteln ist in den letzten Jahren erheblich vergrößert worden. Die richtige Lagerung dieser Lebensmittel und sachkundige Beratung der Kunden setzt beim Fachverkäufer eine gute Warenkenntnis voraus. Eine Warenkunde für diese spezifische Lebensmittelgruppe gab es bisher nicht. Diese Lücke wurde mit dem vorliegenden Buch geschlossen. Neben der warenkundlichen Betrachtung von kalorienreduzierten Lebensmitteln, von Säuglings- und Kleinkindernahrung, Diabetiker-Lebensmitteln, diätetischen Lebensmitteln für spezielle Erkrankungen und von Gesundheitspflegemitteln sind in besonderen Kapiteln in komprimierter Form u. a. die allgemeinen ernährungsphysiologischen Grundlagen einer gesunden Ernährung, die diätetischen Grundlagen zur Vorbeugung, Behandlung und Nachbehandlung einiger wichtiger Krankheitsgruppen, Grundkenntnisse über Qualitätssicherung im

Handel, die planmäßige Gestaltung der Warenfonds und die Aufgaben des Groß- und Einzelhandels bei der weiteren Durchsetzung einer gesunden Ernährung dargestellt. Damit rundet sich das Buch zu einem ausgezeichneten Hilfsmittel für die Berufsausbildung von Fachverkäufern und für Studierende ab, es ist ein vorzüglicher Berater für die im Lebensmittelhandel und an allen anderen Stellen der Volksernährung Tätigen.

Ein Verzeichnis von Begriffen aus dem Bereich der Medizin, Ernährungsphysiologie und Lebensmittelchemie mit Erläuterungen, ein Literaturverzeichnis sowie ein Sachwortverzeichnis erleichtern die Arbeit mit dem Buch. Bedauert werden muß, daß es nicht möglich war, die zur gleichen Zeit veröffentlichten neuen Durchschnittswerte für den Energie- und Nährstoffbedarf anstelle der veralteten Empfehlungen aus dem Jahre 1969 in Tabelle 1 aufzunehmen. M. ZOBEL

N. D. PINTAURO: TEA AND SOLUBLE TEA PRODUCTS MANUFACTURE. 261 Seiten, 31 Abb. Noyes Data Corporation, Park Ridge, New Jersey, USA, 1977, Preis: 32,— $.

Wie für zahlreiche andere Lebensmittel, liegt nun auch für Tee und seine Verarbeitungsprodukte eine systematische, die letzten 20 Jahre umfassende Patentsammlung vor. Damit wird der wachsenden Bedeutung dieses Getränkes Rechnung getragen, dessen Konsum zwar z. B. in den USA mengenmäßig hinter Kaffee, Milch, alkoholfreien Erfrischungsgetränken und Fruchtsäften erst an 5. Stelle rangiert, das zugleich aber mit 8% jährlicher Zuwachsrate die höchste Verbrauchssteigerung aufweist.

Neue Patente zur Teeverarbeitung und -zubereitung betreffen im wesentlichen 4 Einsatzgebiete: die Verarbeitung von Teeblättern zu schwarzem Tee einschließlich von Welk-, Sortier- und Fermentationsprozessen, die Extraktion und Konzentrierung, die Aromaerhaltung und Aromatisierung sowie die Vereinfachung der Zubereitung durch Einsatz von Teebeuteln.

Der Band stellt keine kritische Sichtung des vorhandenen Materials dar, sondern nur eine registrierende Patentsammlung. Durch Reduktion des Inhalts der einzelnen Patente auf das Wesentliche und eine Einführung in die jeweiligen Hauptkapitel wird aber die Gewinnung eines Überblicks über die Patentsituation sehr erleichtert. Einziger Nachteil ist die alleinige Berücksichtigung amerikanischer und englischer Patente. Wenn auch die wichtigen europäischen, sowjetischen und japanischen Patente in der Mehrzahl der Fälle zugleich in den USA angemeldet worden sind, so wird doch eine aufwendige Ergänzung überall dort notwendig, wo ein lückenloser Überblick erforderlich ist. M. ROTHE

N. P. KOSMINA: BIOCHEMIE DER BROTHERSTELLUNG, (Übersetzung aus dem Russischen) 392 Seiten, 136 Abb., 200 Tab. VEB Fachbuchverlag, Leipzig 1977, Preis: 43,80 M (DDR); 54,— (Ausland).

Der wissenschaftliche und technologische Stand de Brotherstellung befindet sich gegenwärtig in einem Übergangsstadium. Bisherige überwiegend auf Empirie beruhende Erfahrungen werden zunehmend durch experimentell gesicherte Kenntnisse ersetzt, die zugleich den Weg zu teil- bzw. vollautomatisierten Technologien öffnen. Die bekannte sowjetische Autorin legt diesen Gesichtspunkt ihrer Monographie zugrunde. Es werden behandelt: die Rohstoffe Weizen und Roggen, ihre Inhaltsstoffe, insbesondere die Rolle der Eiweißkomponenten bei der Teigherstellung unter Berücksichtigung von Gärung, Mikroflora des Mehles, Gärungsmikroorganismen und Backprozeß. Enthalten sind ferner Kapitel mit Beschreibungen wichtiger Untersuchungsverfahren, Methoden zur Qualitätsverbesserung von Mehlen, der Regulierung der Enzymaktivität durch Einsatz mikrobieller bzw. pflanzlicher Enzyme sowie der Verwendung von oberflächenaktiven Stoffen und chemischen Verbesserungsmitteln. Da das im Literaturverzeichnis (31 S.) ausgewertete Schrifttum nur bis etwa 1969 reicht, ist der neueste Erkenntnisstand des in rascher Entwicklung befindlichen Gebietes leider nicht berücksichtigt. Das ist sicher mit ein Grund dafür, warum im Vergleich zu den Eiweißstoffen die Kohlenhydrate und ihre Wechselwirkungen, aber auch die Aromaproblematik zu knapp abgehandelt sind. Einige im Zusammenhang mit der Übersetzung verbundene Unstimmigkeiten sollten, das sei bei einer vorgesehenen Neuauflage empfohlen, korrigiert werden: beispielsweise die Angabe von Buchtiteln in der Originalsprache, die Eliminierung des Begriffes „Milchmolke“ und die Veränderung der Bezeichnung „Präferment“ durch den gebräuchlicheren Begriff „Vorgäransatz“. Die Autorin hat eine gute Grundlage geschaffen, die aber inzwischen einer Aktualisierung bedarf. A. TÄUFEL

M. H. GUTCHO: FREEZE DRYING PROCESSES FOR THE FOOD INDUSTRY. IX und 400 Seiten. 109 Abb., 192 Patentnachweise. Noyes Data Corporation, Park Ridge, New Jersey, USA, 1977. Preis: 39,— $.

Die Gefriertrocknung ist zweifellos die beste Art zur Gewinnung hochwertiger Trockenlebensmittel. Ihre Einsatzfähigkeit wird jedoch durch hohe Kosten und lange Trocknungszeiten erheblich eingeschränkt. Am US-amerikanischen Patentschrifttum der Jahre 1961 bis 1975 wird aufgezeigt, welche technischen Neuerungen und Verbesserungen der jüngsten Zeit das Verfahren weniger kostenintensiv und für die Lebensmittelindustrie praxisreifer machen können. In 3 Hauptkapiteln (Durchführung der Gefriertrocknung, Ausrüstungen zur Gefriertrocknung, Gefriertrocknung spezieller Lebensmittel) werden die verschiedenen Arten der Gefriertechnik, Hitzetransfermechanismen, Sublimation, Enteisung sowie Kontrolle und Steuerung des Verfahrens, neue Anlagen, Ausrüstungselemente und Arbeitsweisen, insbesondere zur Verkürzung und kontinuierlichen Gestaltung der Verfahrensabläufe und zur Kostenreduzierung sowie Möglichkeiten der Prozeßgestaltung zur Trocknung von Kaffee, Tee, Fleisch- und Milchprodukten, Gemüse, Früchten, Säften und anderen Erzeugnissen der Lebensmittelindustrie aufgezeigt. Das Buch bietet eine Fülle technischer Detaileinsichten. Aus den auf Grund ihrer Zweckbestimmung nicht leicht überschaubaren Patentschriften hebt es das Wesentliche der Verfahrensführungen, -prinzipien und -techniken heraus und ermöglicht so eine schnelle Information über den technischen Fortschritt auf diesem Gebiet. Für die erfaßten Patente sind am Ende Autoren-, Firmen- und Patentnummernregister zusammengestellt. B. GASSMANN

Die Nahrung 22, 3 (1978) K9 - K11

Zentralinstitut für Ernährung in Potsdam-Rehbrücke
(Direktor: Prof.Dr. H.Haenel), Forschungszentrum für
Molekularbiologie und Medizin, Akademie der Wissenschaften
der DDR

FRAKTIONIERUNG VON OLIGO-GALAKTURONSÄUREN AN DEAE-CELLULOSE

(Wissenschaftlicher Kurzbericht)

H. Anger und M. Krause

Für die Untersuchung des enzymatischen Pektinsäure- bzw. Pektinabbaus sowie für die Isolierung bestimmter Abbauprodukte ist die genaue Kenntnis der qualitativen und quantitativen Zusammensetzung der Oligomeren in entsprechenden Hydrolysaten eine notwendige Voraussetzung. Im folgenden wird der Einfluß der Molmasse des Pektins auf die Fraktionierung an DEAE-Cellulose [1] zur Auftrennung der Galakturonsäure-Oligomeren in mit Endo-Polygalakturonase (EC 3.2.1.15.) aus Aspergillus spec. [2] erhaltenen Pektinsäurehydrolysaten ausgenutzt.

An einer 2x6-cm-Säule aus DEAE-Cellulose (Schleicher & Schüll) gelingt durch Aufbau eines gekrümmten Gradienten (Abb.1, unten) zwischen 0,002 M Dinatriumhydrogenphosphat/0,001 M EDTA (pH 6,5) und 0,20 M Dinatriumhydrogenphosphat/0,001 M EDTA (pH 6,5) die Fraktionierung der Galakturonsäure-Oligomeren über den bisher bekannten Bereich des Polymerisationsgrades $P \leq 5$ an Sephadex G 25 [3] bzw. $P \leq 9$ an DEAE-Sephadex [4] hinaus. Der Nachweis erfolgt in den einzelnen Fraktionen über die Phenol-Schwefelsäure-Reaktion [5]. Der anfangs steile und zunehmend flacher werdende Verlauf des Gradienten wird aus der Abhängigkeit des Polymerisationsgrades von der Pufferkonzentration bei linearem Gradientenverlauf entnommen. Ein auf diese Weise erhaltenes Chromatogramm wird in Abb.1 (oben) dargestellt. Es kann eine Auftrennung der Galakturonsäure-Oligomeren bis P = 15 erreicht werden. Die weiteren Fraktionen im Chromatogramm stellen Gemische dar; sie entstehen durch stufenweise Elution mit 0,25 M Dinatriumhydrogenphosphat/0,001 M EDTA (pH 6,5) und 0,1 N Natronlauge.

Trägt man den Polymerisationsgrad gegen die Fraktionsnummer auf, so ergibt sich die in Abb.2 wiedergegebene lineare Beziehung.

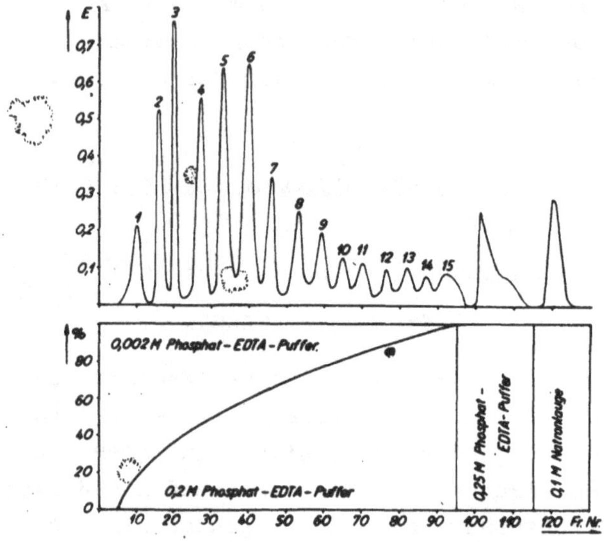

Abb.1. Auftrennung der nach Polygalakturonase-Abbau (EC 3.2.1.15.) von Citruspektinsäure erhaltenen Galakturonsäure-Oligomeren an DEAE-Cellulose (oben); Gradientenverlauf und Elutionsmittelfolge (unten)

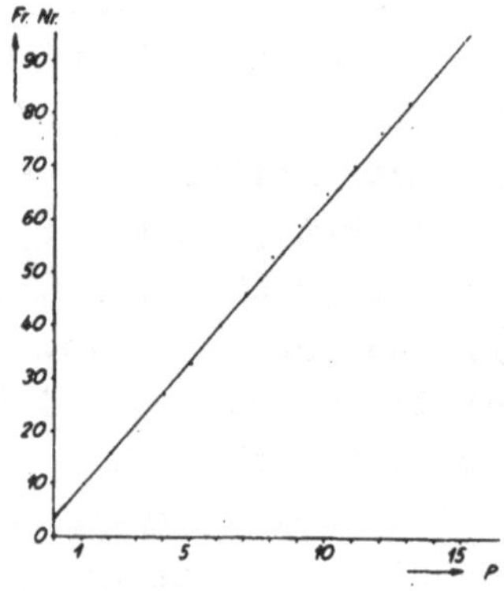

Abb.2. Abhängigkeit der Fraktionsnummer (Fr.-Nr.) vom Polymerisationsgrad (P) der Galakturonsäure-Oligomeren

Für jeden Polymerisationsgrad stehen demnach durchschnittlich 6 Fraktionen zur Verfügung. Für die präparative Fraktionierung der Oligo-Galakturonsäuren empfiehlt es sich, die Dauer des Gradientendurchlaufs auf 48 h zu verlängern, so daß die Anzahl der Fraktionen für jeden Polymerisationsgrad entsprechend zunimmt.

L i t e r a t u r

[1] Anger, H., R. Friebe u. G. Dongowski, Nahrung 21, 731 (1977).

[2] Bock, W., M. Krause, H. Göbel, H. Anger, H.-J. Schawaller, Ch.Flemming u.A. Gabert, Nahrung 22, 183 (1978).

[3] Rexová-Benková, L., Chem. zvesti 24, 59 (1970).

[4] Hatanaka, C., u.J. Ozawa, Nippon Nogei Kagaku Kaishi 46, 417 (1972); ref.in C.A. 78, 72 501 (1973).

[5] Dubois, M., K.A. Gilles, J.K. Hamilton, P.A. Rebers u. F. Smith, Analyt.Chem. 28, 350 (1956).

Dr. H.Anger und Dr. M.Krause, Zentralinstitut für Ernährung, DDR-1505 Bergholz-Rehbrücke, Arthur-Scheunert-Allee 114-116

Eingegangen 20.2.1978

Die Nahrung 22, 3 (1978) K13 - K15

Zentralinstitut für Ernährung in Potsdam-Rehbrücke (Direktor: Prof.Dr. H.Haenel), Forschungszentrum für Molekularbiologie und Medizin, Akademie der Wissenschaften der DDR, und Hygieneinstitut des Bezirkes Potsdam (Ärztlicher Direktor: MR Dr.H. Ritschel)

ZUM VORKOMMEN VON TOXISCHEN SCHWERMETALLEN (CADMIUM, BLEI, ZINK UND QUECKSILBER) IN PILZEN

(Wissenschaftlicher Kurzbericht)

H. Woggon und K. Bickerich

Seit einiger Zeit mehren sich in der Literatur Hinweise auf höhere Gehalte von Cadmium und Quecksilber in Speisepilzen. Besondere Aufmerksamkeit erregten die hohen Cadmium- und Quecksilberkonzentrationen bei bestimmten wildwachsenden Champignonarten. Dieses aktuelle Problem war Anlaß zu einigen gezielten Schwermetallbestimmungen, insbesondere am wildwachsenden Schafchampignon. Von Interesse war dabei ein Vergleich mit Zuchtchampignons und einigen anderen Pilzarten.

Die analysierten Pilze wurden zwischen Oktober und Dezember 1976 bzw. 1977 im Raum Potsdam gesammelt bzw. aus Pilzzüchtereien im Raum Berlin entnommen. Vor der Untersuchung wurden die Pilze küchenmäßig vorbereitet, so daß nur die genußfähigen und gewaschenen Anteile zur Untersuchung gelangten. Alle Metallgehalte beziehen sich auf Trockengewichte. Der Aufschluß der bei 80 °C getrockneten Proben erfolgte durch Trockenveraschung bei 450 °C. Cadmium, Blei und Zink wurden nach Extraktion mit Diäthylammoniumdiäthyldithiocarbamat in Butylacetat mittels Atomabsorptionsspektrophotometrie (AAS 1 des VEB Carl Zeiß, Jena) in der Flamme bestimmt. Die Bestimmung des Quecksilbers erfolgte nach Säureaufschluß durch Atomabsorption nach dem Kaltdampfverfahren.

Ergebnis

In Tab.1 sind die gefundenen Schwermetallgehalte zusammengestellt. Deutlich erkennbar ist der große Unterschied im Cadmiumgehalt von Schafchampignon (Ø 32,2 mg/kg) und Zuchtchampignon (Ø 0,30 mg/kg). Auch gegenüber dem Straßenegerling (Agaricus bitorquis) ergibt sich ein 10fach höherer Cadmiumgehalt. Bei Quecksilber werden signifikant höhere Gehalte im Schafchampignon (5:1) gefunden. Deutlich höher sind auch die Bleiwerte. Im

Tabelle 1

Cd-, Pb-, Zn- und Hg-Gehalte in Pilzen [mg/kg Trockensubstanz]

Pilzart	Cd	Pb	Zn	Hg
Schafchampignon Agaricus arvensis	28,4 28,4 39,7	4,1 3,45 2,84	-+) -+) 399,0	4,14 3,28 1,40
Straßenegerling Agaricus bitorquis	3,75	6,05	143,3	3,33
Violetter Rötelritterling Lepista nuda	1,40	4,20	147,0	2,57
Lilastieliger Rötelritterling Lepista personata	1,07	3,10	151,0	4,42
Knäul-Ritterling Lyophyllum conglobatum	1,15	3,10	83,5	0,24
Austernseitling (Zucht) Pleurotus ostreatus	0,70	1,95	115,5	0,19
Zuchtchampignon Agaricus bisporus				
Pilzzüchterei Fuhl/Falkensee	0,63 0,22	1,95 1,61	92,5 67,5	0,06 - +)
Pilzzucht Rehbrücke	0,10	0,35	-+)	0,15
Pilzzucht Kleintierhaltung Falkensee	0,18	0,75	-+)	0,58
Pilzzüchterei LPG 1.Mai Wartenberg-Lindenberg	0,26	1,34	47,2	1,14
VEG Champignon-Zucht Berlin-Biesdorf	0,43	2,04	58,0	0,76

-+) Analysen nicht durchgeführt

Vergleich zu den in Lebensmitteln üblicherweise vorkommenden Bleigehalten sind diese jedoch nur mäßig erhöht. In den Zuchtchampignons liegen die Gehalte an Blei, Cadmium, Zink und Quecksilber in einer Größenordnung, wie sie bei Lebensmitteln im allgemeinen vorkommen. Der sehr hohe Bleiwert beim Straßenegerling (Entfernung von einer Hauptverkehrsstraße 1 m) deutet vielleicht auf eine erhöhte Umweltkontamination durch Kraftfahrzeugabgase hin.

Die Toleranzgrenzen werden nur beim Cd vom Schafchampignon überschritten, und zwar um das Fünf- bis Zehnfache. Die höheren Cd-Konzentrationen liegen somit in der gleichen Größenordnung, wie sie auch von einigen anderen Autoren [1,2] - ebenfalls an sehr unterschiedlichen Standorten - bei der Art Agaricus arvensis gefunden wurden. Das gleiche trifft für den Quecksilbergehalt zu. Auch Woidich u.a. [4], Seeger [5] und Aichberger [3] stellten verhältnismäßig hohe Quecksilberkonzentrationen in einigen Champignonarten fest.

Es stellt sich somit die Frage, worauf diese Unterschiede zurückzuführen sind. Nach Untersuchungen von Meisch [1] konnten standortbedingte Einflüsse wie höherer Boden-Cd-Gehalt nicht nachgewiesen werden. Vielmehr deutet vieles darauf hin, daß hier art- oder auch rassenbedingte, für Cadmium spezifische Aufnahme- und Bindungsmechanismen bestehen.

Welche möglichen toxischen Konsequenzen ergeben sich aus dem wiederholten Verzehr solcher Cd-reichen Pilze? Vergleicht man die von der WHO tolerierte Grenzdosis von 0,5 mg Cd/Woche mit der einer Champignonmahlzeit von 1 kg Frischgewicht (etwa 100 g Trockengewicht), so ergibt sich bei einer einzigen Mahlzeit für den Schafchampignon eine mindestens 5fache Überschreitung des o. g. Toleranzwertes, die jedoch noch keine Gefährdung der Gesundheit bedeutet. Solange aber ausreichende Informationen über Resorption und Metabolisierung der Cd-Verbindungen aus den Pilzen nicht vorliegen, muß vor einem übermäßigen kontinuierlichen Genuß bestimmter Champignonarten, insbesondere des Schafchampignons, gewarnt werden.

Literatur

[1] Meisch, H.-U., I.A. Schmitt u. W.Reinle, Z.Naturforsch. 32c, 172 (1977).

[2] Collet, P., Dt.Lebensmittel-Rdsch. 73, 75 (1977).

[3] Aichberger, K., Z.Lebensmittel-Untersuch.u.-Forsch. 163, 35 (1977).

[4] Woidich, H., u.W. Pfannhauser, Dt.Lebensmittel-Rdsch. 71, 177 (1975).

[5] Seeger, R., Z.Lebensmittel-Untersuch.u.-Forsch. 161, 115 (1976).

Dr.H. Woggon, Zentralinstitut für Ernährung, DDR-1505 Bergholz-Rehbrücke, Arthur-Scheunert-Allee 114-116

Eingegangen 24.2.1978

CONTENTS

СОДЕРЖАНИЕ

INHALTSVERZEICHNIS

Bezugsmöglichkeiten:

Bestellungen sind zu richten

in der DDR an eine Buchhandlung oder an den Akademie-Verlag,
DDR-108 Berlin, Leipziger Straße 3–4

im sozialistischen Ausland an eine Buchhandlung für fremdsprachige Literatur oder an den zuständigen Postzeitungsvertrieb

in der BRD und Westberlin an eine Buchhandlung oder an die Auslieferungsstelle
KUNST UND WISSEN, Erich Bieber,
7 Stuttgart 1, Wilhelmstraße 4–6

in Österreich an den Globus-Buchvertrieb,
1201 Wien, Höchstädtplatz 3

im übrigen Ausland an den Internationalen Buch- und Zeitschriftenhandel; den Buchexport, Volkseigener Außenhandelsbetrieb der Deutschen Demokratischen Republik,
DDR-701 Leipzig, Postfach 160, oder
an den Akademie-Verlag
DDR-108 Berlin, Leipziger Straße 3–4

FSC
www.fsc.org
MIX
Papier | Fördert
gute Waldnutzung
FSC® C083411

Zeitfracht Medien GmbH
Ferdinand-Jühlke-Straße 7
99095 Erfurt, Deutschland
produktsicherheit@kolibri360.de